The Ethics of Pandemics

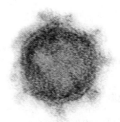

The Ethics of Pandemics

EDITED BY MEREDITH CELENE SCHWARTZ

broadview press

BROADVIEW PRESS – www.broadviewpress.com
Peterborough, Ontario, Canada

Founded in 1985, Broadview Press remains a wholly independent publishing house. Broadview's focus is on academic publishing; our titles are accessible to university and college students as well as scholars and general readers. With 800 titles in print, Broadview has become a leading international publisher in the humanities, with world-wide distribution. Broadview is committed to environmentally responsible publishing and fair business practices.

Library and Archives Canada Cataloguing in Publication

Title: The ethics of pandemics / edited by Meredith Celene Schwartz.
Names: Schwartz, Meredith Celene, editor.
Description: Includes bibliographical references and index.
Identifiers: Canadiana (print) 20200275127 | Canadiana (ebook) 20200275194 |
    ISBN 9781554815449 (softcover) | ISBN 9781770487680 (PDF) | ISBN 9781460407202
    (EPUB)
Subjects: LCSH: COVID-19 (Disease)—Moral and ethical aspects—Textbooks. | LCSH: Epidemics—
    Moral and ethical aspects—Textbooks. | LCSH: Public health—Moral and ethical aspects—
    Textbooks. | LCGFT: Textbooks.
Classification: LCC RA644.C67 E84 2020 | DDC 362.1962/414—dc23

Broadview Press handles its own distribution in North America:
PO Box 1243, Peterborough, Ontario K9J 7H5, Canada
555 Riverwalk Parkway, Tonawanda, NY 14150, USA
Tel: (705) 743-8990; Fax: (705) 743-8353
email: customerservice@broadviewpress.com

For all territories outside of North America, distribution is handled by Eurospan Group.

Broadview Press acknowledges the financial support of the Government of Canada for our publishing activities.

Canada

Edited by Martin R. Boyne

Book design by Chris Rowat Design

PRINTED IN CANADA

Contents

Introduction

I began collecting articles for this book in mid-January 2020. It was the Lunar New Year in the year of the Earth Rat. Chinese astrologers predicted that "the Year of the Gengzi," which comes once every 60 years, would be a bad one for global politics and the economy.[1] The radio was reporting that China had extended its new year's celebrations to control the spread of a new virus. By the end of January, China had begun to build a new hospital to treat coronavirus patients. They said they would complete construction in ten days. It seemed to me that this virus was something to keep an eye on.

At first there were few reports and many rumors about what was happening in Wuhan. By the end of January there was some discussion of the ethical issues arising in the context of the novel coronavirus, but it remained sparse.[2] Mid-February, the World Health Organization released a report about the infectious virus.[3] The English-language medical journals I was reading (the *Journal of the American Medical Association* [JAMA], the *New England Journal of Medicine* [NEJM], the *British Medical Journal* [BMJ], and the *Canadian Medical Association Journal* [CMAJ]) were largely silent, with only a few reports from Chinese doctors. Then as February turned to March and COVID-19 cases began to affect Europe and North America, there came a torrent of information. Nearly every article published in the medical journals focused on COVID-19. The pace of research accelerated, with labs cooperating across the globe. Whereas at the beginning of the pandemic it was difficult to find reliable information, by March it was hard to keep up with the many articles that were being released, most of them in pre-print form pending peer review.

To compile the readings in this book, I read over 700 academic articles along with countless news pieces, selecting some of the best among them. As the majority of the included articles were written in the spring of 2020, at a time when the long-term effects of COVID-19 were very much uncertain, it's unavoidable that some aspects will be dated soon after publication. Statistics and other factual claims are reflective of the data available at the time of each reading's composition, and since many of these details change on a daily basis, it's not possible to offer more than a "snapshot" of what is known or believed at a particular point. The immediate relevance of the issues addressed in this text may also shift over time, depending in part on how governments, health-care researchers, and society respond to these challenges. Other important ethical and political issues may arise as well in the coming years.

Nonetheless, we can be certain that many of the core ethical issues and arguments addressed in this book will be relevant in future health crises, even if some of the details differ. Continuing to study and reflect on these topics will make us better prepared, whether in connection with a pandemic comparable to COVID-19 or in response to other disasters, be they global or local. Many of these ethical concerns apply outside of a crisis situation. Even at times of prosperity, it matters how we allocate health-care resources among the population, how we conceive of the obligations of health-care professionals and our obligations toward them, and how we reflect on racial disparities in health outcomes.

Because of the constraints we faced in producing this book quickly and in the midst of a pandemic, I had to make some difficult choices about what to include. As a result, many important topics have unfortunately been left out. For example, the book does not have a reading on how the pandemic is affecting men and women differently. In some countries, like the United Kingdom, men seem to be dying more frequently from COVID-19,[4] although women have been more likely to contract the virus in Canada.[5] As this is the first service-driven economic recession and women are more likely to work in the service industry, women's earnings have taken a bigger hit than men's.[6] Schools, nurseries, and daycares are closed, and children are learning from home, forcing parents to make hard decisions about how they will cover childcare. Women have disproportionately shouldered this added childcare labor. This is in part due to entrenched social roles, but it is also because women are paid less on average, so many mothers have temporarily left their jobs while fathers have stayed at their higher wage positions so as to retain the greatest amount of household income.[7] The effects of this disparity can be seen in many areas, including academia, where women have been submitting fewer articles and taking on fewer projects than their male peers.[8] Though the provided articles say little about the unique effects the pandemic has had on women, I have integrated broader considerations of equity throughout. Inequities have touched every aspect of the pandemic response and are apparent at both the domestic and the global levels.

The effects of COVID-related shutdowns on non-human animals constitute another important topic that the book does not cover. Those effects are varied: some animals are thriving with less human presence to disturb them,[9] while others have suffered from an increase in poaching.[10] Although many animal shelters were emptied early in the pandemic by people working from home and seeking comfort and distraction, as the pandemic has worn on other pets have been euthanized or sent to shelters as their humans have died from the disease.[11] Having seen the speed at which COVID-19 infections have torn through the meat industry, more people have also begun to rethink our food systems and our reliance on other animals.[12]

The book also does not cover any of the beneficial aspects of the pandemic; although it's easy to lose sight of these amidst all of the bad news, there have been a few good outcomes too. Daily CO_2 emissions went down as much as 26% at the height of the shutdowns.[13] Many people have enjoyed spending extra time with their families or taking advantage of travel restrictions and reduced commutes to read books, watch shows, and take on creative projects that they've previously put off. Working from home also offers the ability to work in one's pajamas; there's a running joke that many of us are wearing business outfits on top and only underwear on the bottom. For many of us, the pandemic has also afforded time to reflect on our societies and health-care systems, and on how they might be improved upon reopening.

Our hope is that this book will offer a unique glimpse into how our society has responded to a disaster that is complex and rapidly changing. Though dangerous pandemics have occurred at various points in human history, COVID-19 has caught many of us off-guard and has entailed the use of protective measures such as border closures and severe travel restrictions that seemed out of the question even as the virus began its spread. It would be inaccurate to say that there weren't some well-informed and perceptive scientists, philosophers, and other experts who predicted the occurrence of a pandemic of this scale. But nonetheless, the published literature on the ethics of pandemics prior to COVID-19 was limited and didn't reflect the full range of issues that have now become so prominent. The rapidity of the virus's spread has in some ways forced academics and other policy thinkers out of their comfort zone, as the need for urgent action has required research, reflection, and publication at extraordinary speed. The readings included in this volume reflect some of the best efforts of philosophers, health-care experts, journalists, and others to synthesize existing literature with the novel features of a pressing public health disaster. In that sense, this book may offer a glimpse into how we as a people reasoned and reacted to one crisis, which may make us better informed in the face of future crises.

We hope that you stay healthy and well informed.

We've created a website containing links to a curated selection of additional readings addressing the issues covered in this book as well as other related topics such as racial bigotry and non-human animals. This website will be updated regularly and can be freely accessed at the address below.

sites.broadviewpress.com/pandemics/

Please note that, while the majority of texts included in this anthology are provided in their entirety, some have been edited for length. Additionally, because some of the included readings were originally published online, with hyperlinks used for citations and references, some formatting modifications have been made in order to offer these readings in print form. Where appropriate, endnote references have been added to the readings to indicate the linked sources of quotations, statistics, and other important facts.

NOTES

1 Joanna Chiu (6 March 2020), "War, Famine...Coronavirus? Chinese Astrologers Prophesied a 'Year of Doom' in 2020," *Toronto Star*.

2 Ruipeng Lei and Renzong Qiu (31 January 2020), "Report from China: Ethical Questions on the Response to the Coronavirus," *The Hastings Center Bioethics Forum*. [blog]

3 World Health Organization (WHO) (16–24 February 2020), *Report of the WHO-China Joint Mission on Coronavirus Disease 2019 (COVID-19)*.

4 Annie Campbell and Sarah Caul (15 May 2020), "Deaths Involving COVID-19, England and Wales: Deaths Occurring in April 2020," *Office for National Statistics*.

5 Jean-Paul R. Soucy and Isha Berry, with contributions from Matthew T. Warkentin and Jens von Bergmann and the COVID-19 Canada Open Data Working Group "COVID-19 in Canada," *The University of Toronto Dalla Lana School of Public Health*, https://art-bd.shinyapps.io/covid19canada/.

6 Armine Yalnizyan (9 April 2020), "COVID-19's Impact: Not Recession but a Completely Different Economics," *Toronto Star*.

7 Helen Lewis (19 March 2020), "The Coronavirus Is a Disaster for Feminism: Pandemics Affect Men and Women Differently," *The Atlantic*.

8 Giuliana Viglione (20 May 2020), "Are Women Publishing Less during the Pandemic? Here's What the Data Say," *Nature*.

9 Jason G. Goldman (21 May 2020), "How the Coronavirus Has Changed Animals' Landscape of Fear," *Scientific American*.

10 Alexander Matthews (20 May 2020), "The Wild Animals at Risk in Lockdown," *Future Planet*.

11 Kara Scannell (12 May 2020), "This Is What Happens to the Pets Left Behind When Their Owners Die from Coronavirus," *CNN*.

12 Gene Baur (19 May 2020), "It's Time to Dismantle Factory Farms and Get Used to Eating Less Meat," *The Guardian*.

13 Corinne Le Quéré et al. (19 May, 2020), "Temporary Reduction in Daily Global CO_2 Emissions during the COVID-19 Forced Confinement," *Nature Climate Change*.

1
Public Health Ethics

INTRODUCTION

The early days of bioethics, in the 1960s and 1970s, were dominated by concerns about clinical medicine and research ethics. The ethical approaches that were developed in that context tended to focus on individual patients and research participants.

More recently, bioethicists have paid increasing attention to public health ethics, especially following the SARS near-pandemic in 2002–03. Whereas clinical medicine focuses on the health of individuals, public health focuses on protecting and promoting the health of populations. There is currently no consensus as to which theory or moral approach is best suited to the advancement of public health. A traditional individualist approach would understand the issues of public health to involve balancing the rights and liberties of persons against the achievement of good health outcomes for the population as a whole. A more relational approach to public health ethics draws attention to social injustices such as racial and class inequality, which often have significant bearing on the health outcomes of members of different populations.[1]

In this chapter, John Authers uses Rawlsian, utilitarian, libertarian, and communitarian approaches to assess various aspects of the COVID-19 pandemic. The majority of the moral perspectives that Authers discusses adopt an individualistic approach to public health ethics. In contrast, Nuala Kenny, Susan Sherwin, and Françoise Baylis endorse a relational approach through which we are encouraged to consider how existing inequalities within society are frequently exacerbated during crises such as pandemics.

1

KEY TERMS

autonomy: comes from the Greek for "self-rule." Autonomy entails that patients who have the capacity to make medical decisions for themselves have a right to do so, and these decisions must be respected by health-care professionals.

COVID-19: an abbreviation for "Coronavirus Disease 2019." This disease is caused by the coronavirus known as SARS-CoV-2. The World Health Organization (WHO) declared COVID-19 to be a pandemic on March 11, 2020.

epidemic: an infectious disease that is spread rapidly and causes illness (morbidity) and death (mortality) across a substantial portion of the population.

pandemic: a worldwide epidemic.

SARS-CoV-2: an abbreviation for "Severe Acute Respiratory Syndrome Coronavirus 2." SARS-CoV-2 is the virus that causes the COVID-19 disease.

NOTE

1 Madison Powers and Ruth Faden, *Social Justice: The Moral Foundations of Public Health and Health Policy* (New York: Oxford University Press, 2006).

1.1

How Coronavirus Is Shaking Up the Moral Universe
The Pandemic Is Putting Profound Philosophical Questions to the Test

John Authers

The coronavirus pandemic is a test. It's a test of medical capacity and political will. It's a test of endurance and forbearance, for believers a test of religious faith. It's a test, too, of a different kind of faith, in the strength of the ideas humans choose to help them form moral judgments and guide personal and social behavior.

The epidemic forces everyone to confront deep questions of human existence, questions so profound that they have previously been answered, in many different ways, by the greatest philosophers. It's a test of where all humans stand.

What is right and what is wrong? What can individuals expect from society, and what can society expect of them? Should others make sacrifices for me, and vice versa? Is it just to set economic limits to fighting a deadly disease?

The lieutenant governor of Texas thinks that those over 70 "shouldn't sacrifice the country" by shutting down economic activity, but should instead be ready to sacrifice themselves. A 22-year-old partying on Spring break in Florida becomes a social media sensation with a different critique of social distancing, saying, "If I get corona, I get corona." Consciously or not, both men are placing themselves in distinct moral traditions.

Several philosophies of social justice have claimed wide adherence in the modern world. They do not line up neatly with party political labels, and most people have sympathy for more than one. Here is a guide to some of the leading idea systems undergirding competing conceptions of right and wrong. Each is being put to the test. As you are put to the test, which do you choose?

Rawlsians

Many westerners are Rawlsians without knowing it. Fifty years ago, the Harvard philosopher John Rawls tried to work out how people would construct their society if the choice had to be made behind what he called a "veil of ignorance" about whether they will be rich, poor or somewhere in-between. Faced with the risk of being the worst off, Rawls posited, humans would not demand total equality, but would need to be assured of the trappings of a modern welfare state. The assurance of basic necessities and the opportunity to do better would form the foundation for social and political justice and provide the ability for people to assert themselves.

Rawls's monumental 1971 book, *A Theory of Justice*, is now regarded as the clearest moral and intellectual justification for modern center-left mixed economies. But the idea comes from somewhere deeper. Rawls was not religious, but his philosophy is essentially in line with the golden rule handed down by the Old Testament prophets and by Jesus, that we should do as we would want to be done by. Some religious leaders have approached the awful dilemmas presented by the coronavirus just as Rawls would, by taking treatment of the worst off as the criterion for social action.

"I hope the lessons we take from our country's experience with COVID-19 aren't about food or avoiding the spread of germs," wrote Russell Moore, the president of the Ethics and Religious Liberty Commission of the Southern Baptist Convention, in the *New York Times*, "but about how we treat the most vulnerable among us. A pandemic is no time to turn our eyes away from the sanctity of human life."[1]

Pope Francis also invoked sympathy for the most afflicted as he addressed a prayer to an empty St. Peter's Square. "We have realized that we are on the same boat, all of us fragile and disoriented, but at the same time important and needed, all of us called to row together, each of us in need of comforting the other," he said.[2]

Perhaps because of their religious resonance, Rawlsian ideas have guided the approach to the pandemic chosen by authorities in the western world. Societies are mobilizing, and governments are taking extra powers to mandate claustrophobic lockdowns in a bid to minimize the death and suffering of the weakest.

Even those who aren't religious tend to accept the logic of the veil of ignorance. If a person is unwilling to be abandoned, governments are not entitled to give up on them; they must do their best to protect everyone, particularly the weakest.

Utilitarians

Other philosophies produce very different ways of dealing with the epidemic. Under utilitarianism, most associated with the nineteenth-century British philosopher John Stuart Mill, rulers must be guided to the total happiness, or "utility," of all the people, and should aim to secure "the greatest good for the greatest number."

In Victorian Britain, this was a radical creed, and the first utilitarians were passionate liberal reformers. But the utilitarian calculus opens up a new possibility—that in situations such as a pandemic, some people might justly be sacrificed for the greater good. It would benefit society to accept casualties, the argument goes, to minimize disruption.

Explicit utilitarian thinking still seems beyond the pale. Last weekend [21–22 March 2020], Britain's *Sunday Times* reported that Dominic Cummings, chief adviser to Prime Minister Boris Johnson, had advocated in private meetings a policy of letting enough people get sick to establish nationwide "herd immunity, protect the economy, and if that means some pensioners die, too bad."[3] It caused an outcry and met with an immediate and impassioned denial by Downing Street. Even Cummings, an iconoclast, refused to be attached to such brutally utilitarian ideas.

Mill himself would not have advocated putting money ahead of people's lives, but a utilitarian calculus is not about balancing money and life. If a recession could lead to shorter lives and widespread misery, it is possible that making less of an attempt to save every last life from the pandemic now could lead to greater total happiness.

In the UK, a paper by an academic at the University of Bristol used mathematical techniques developed to measure the cost-efficiency of safety measures in the nuclear power industry to calculate the likely savings of human life by different approaches to the virus, and found that a 12-month lockdown followed by vaccinations would be best.[4] But it cautioned that this would only create a net saving of life if the reduction in gross domestic product could be kept to 6.4% or less.

That paper, broadcast on the BBC, provoked a fiery response from econo-mists,[5] and some research suggests counterintuitively that recessions lengthen lives.[6] Most people find the mere attempt at such an exercise callous, but it's dif-ficult to dismiss it. Governments and insurers do indeed put a notional price on a human life when setting policy.[7] Must every last patient be given the utmost care if this plan of action causes greater suffering in the long run? Or, as President Donald Trump put it: "We can't have the cure be worse than the problem."[8]

It's intuitive to view moral problems through a utilitarian lens and then to find outcomes like this distasteful, and to reject them because they conflict with the golden rule. If the lockdowns drag on for months, utilitarian ideas may bub-ble back to the surface.

Libertarians

The libertarian place in American thought is long and distinguished. Its lineage goes back at least to the Enlightenment philosopher John Locke and the found-ing fathers, and in its modern incarnation gains inspiration from the author Ayn Rand, who outlined her ideas in novels and essays. For her, man had a right "to live for himself" and an individual's happiness "cannot be prescribed by another man or any number of other men."

The most famous libertarian thought experiment was conducted by another Harvard philosopher, Robert Nozick, in a riposte to Rawls. He imagined what kind of political state would be built, and how much personal liberty citizens would surrender, if everyone were dropped into a utopian landscape with no so-cial structures. The novelist William Golding gave one answer in *The Lord of the Flies*. To avoid the descent into violence that the schoolboys of Golding's novel endure, Nozick, in *Anarchy, State and Utopia*, reckoned that people would set up a very limited state dedicated to self-defense and the protection of individual rights—but nothing more.

The western coronavirus response has hugely expanded state powers and lim-ited individual rights with little debate, and to date populations have consented to privations that Rand and Nozick argued they should never accept.

But wait. There have been objections to lockdowns on the libertarian ba-sis that they infringe on rights. Critiques are appearing saying that politicians haven't proven that such drastic measures are necessary.[9] Before the coronavirus, the US suffered a measles epidemic as the result of anti-vaccination activism, a libertarian cause that put parents' right to choose not to vaccinate their chil-dren above the state's attempt to defend other parents' right to expect that their own children wouldn't have to mix with unvaccinated peers.[10] Panic buying, and hoarding of medical equipment also show that many people are following Rand's idea of self-determination and putting themselves first. Such ideas may grow more appealing after a few more weeks of self-isolation.

In public spaces around the world, libertarians are in conflict with the state. Social media is full of images of big social gatherings, often in luxurious social settings. "If I get corona, I get corona," as the 22-year-old said on video in Florida. "At the end of the day, I'm not gonna let it stop me from partying."[11] Oklahoma's governor even felt the need to tweet that he was at a packed restaurant.

Libertarians are not only found on the political right. As the crisis began to unfold, the American Civil Liberties Union made a statement accepting that civil liberties must "sometimes" give way when it comes to fighting a communicable disease—but "only in ways that are scientifically justified." It said, "The evidence is clear that travel bans and quarantines are not the solution."[12]

The right to walk in a park looks like a flash point. New York Governor Andrew Cuomo was furious to see crowds expressing libertarian sympathies—whether they saw it that way or not—by gathering in parks. "It's arrogant," Cuomo said. "It's self-destructive. It's disrespectful to other people. And it has to stop and it has to stop now!"[13]

New Yorkers are organizing to keep the parks open.[14]

In these conditions, individual choices become freighted with moral significance. How, for example, will society eventually judge behavior like that of Kentucky Senator Rand Paul?[15] Arguably the most prominent libertarian in the US, he continued to socialize as normal for a week after being told that he had had contact with someone who tested positive for the coronavirus. He had no symptoms. Recall that there are many elderly members of the Senate. Last weekend, after a workout in the Senate gym, he discovered that he had himself tested positive.

Communitarians

Yet another approach is based on the notion that everyone derives their identity from the broader community. Individual rights count, but not more than community norms. These notions go back to the Greeks, but in modern times, the philosophy is most widely connected to the sociologist Amitai Etzioni and philosopher Michael Sandel. Sandel's *Liberalism and the Limits of Justice* is another riposte to Rawls, arguing that justice cannot be determined in a vacuum or behind a veil of ignorance, but must be rooted in society. He sets out a theory of justice based on the common good.

Speaking [on 24 March 2020] to Thomas Friedman of the *New York Times*, Sandel said: "The common good is about how we live together in community. It's about the ethical ideals we strive for together, the benefits and burdens we share, the sacrifices we make for one another. It's about the lessons we learn from one another about how to live a good and decent life."[16]

The virus has attacked in exactly this place, depriving everyone of life in a community. And communitarian ideas are showing themselves. Across Europe, people on lockdown have arranged to go to their windows and balconies to applaud their national health services.[17] These are seen as bedrocks of society. At London's Olympic opening ceremony in 2012, a pageant of Britishness, the organizers celebrated the National Health Service with dancing nurses wheeling hospital beds. For many countries with a modern welfare state, celebrating and supporting the workers of their public-health service is seen as a communitarian duty.

This is a critical point of difference with the US, where the expansion of medical care is a hugely contentious issue. Communitarians like Professor Michael Walzer of the Institute for Advanced Study argue that any system of medical provision requires "the constraint of the guild of physicians."[18] The coronavirus promises to bring this debate to a head.

Communitarianism also underlies much social conservative thought. When the very conservative Republican Texas Lieutenant Governor Dan Patrick said on Fox News that the rest of the country should not sacrifice itself for the elderly, he was making a communitarian argument, not a utilitarian one.[19]

"No one reached out to me and said, 'As a senior citizen, are you willing to take a chance on your survival in exchange for keeping the America that all America loves for your children and grandchildren?'" Patrick, who is 63, told the host Tucker Carlson. "And if that's the exchange, I'm all in."

In this telling, it is the patriotic duty of the elderly not to force privations on their country, and make life worse for their grandchildren. Such a communitarian ethic has always resonated within the US (just read Alexis de Tocqueville), and it provoked an outcry on social media.

China practiced another kind of communitarianism after the coronavirus first appeared in Wuhan in January. The people of that city were told to lock themselves in, and often forcibly quarantined, for the good of the community and the state, largely identified with the Communist Party. Under Xi Jinping, the Party has rehabilitated the Confucian thought that long justified obedience to a hierarchical and authoritarian but benevolent state.[20] That the notion of social solidarity remains strong showed in the spectacular discipline with which China and other Asian nations dealt with the problem.

"We Are All Rawlsians Now"

For now, the approach being adopted across the West is Rawlsian. Politicians are working on the assumption that they have a duty to protect everyone as they themselves would wish to be protected, while people are also applying the golden rule as they decide that they should self-isolate for the sake of others. We are all Rawlsians now.

How long will we stay that way? All the other theories of justice have an appeal, and may test the resolve to follow the golden rule. But I suspect that Rawls and the golden rule will win out. That is partly because religion—even if it is in decline in the West—has hard-wired it into our consciousness. And as the

7

epidemic grows worse and brings the disease within fewer degrees of separation for everyone, we may well find that the notion of loving thy neighbor as thyself becomes far more potent.

Notes

1 Russell Moore, "God Doesn't Want Us to Sacrifice the Old," *New York Times*, 26 March 2020.

2 "Pope at Urbi et orbi: Full text of his meditation," *Vatican News*, 27 March 2020.

3 Dominic Cummings, "No 10 denies claim Dominic Cummings argued to 'let old people die,'" *Guardian*, 22 March 2020.

4 Philip Thomas, "J-value assessment of how best to combat COVID-19," *Nanotechnology Perceptions* 16 (2020): 16–40.

5 Jonathan Portes, "Don't believe the myth that we must sacrifice lives to save the economy," *Guardian*, 25 March 2020.

6 Lynne Peeples, "How the next recession could save lives," *Nature*, 23 January 2019.

7 Cass R. Sunstein, "This Time the Numbers Show We Can't Be Too Careful," *Bloomberg*, 26 March 2020.

8 Jill Colvin, Josh Boak, and Ricardo Alonso-Zaldivar, "Trump: 'We Can't Have the Cure Be Worse Than the Problem,'" *Real Clear Politics*, 24 March 2020.

9 John P.A. Ioannidis, "A fiasco in the making? As the coronavirus pandemic takes hold, we are making decisions without reliable data," *STAT*, 17 March 2020; "Why Flattening the Curve Is Overrated," *Pensford Financial*, 23 March 2020.

10 Grace Hauck, "US in danger of losing measles-free status, a 'mortifying' effect of anti-vaxx movement," *USA Today*, 13 September 2019.

11 Aimee Ortiz, "Man Who Said, 'If I Get Corona, I Get Corona,' Apologizes," *New York Times*, 24 March 2020.

12 Jay Stanley, "What You Need to Know about the Coronavirus Outbreak: A Civil Liberties Perspective," *American Civil Liberties Union*, 28 January 2020.

13 Tim Hains, "Cuomo: 'Arrogant,' 'Self-Destructive,' 'Disrespectful' People Not Taking Quarantine Seriously Are 'Making a Mistake,'" *Real Clear Politics*, 22 March 2020.

14 Rose Harvey, "Keep the Parks Open," *City & State NY*, 26 March 2020.

15 Adrianna Rodriguez, "Texas' lieutenant governor suggests grandparents are willing to die for US economy," *USA Today*, 24 March 2020.

16 Thomas L. Friedman, "Finding the 'Common Good' in a Pandemic," *New York Times*, 24 March 2020.

17 Jane Dalton, "Clap for our Carers: UK erupts in applause for NHS workers handling coronavirus crisis," *Independent*, 26 March 2020.

18 Michael Walzer, *Spheres of Justice: A Defense of Pluralism and Equality* (New York: Basic, 1983).

19 Allie Morris and Robert T. Garrett, "Texas Lt. Gov. Dan Patrick spurns shelter in place, urges return to work, suggests grandparents should sacrifice," *Dallas Morning News*, 23 March 2020.

20 H.D.S. Greenway, "China's rehabilitation of Confucius," *Boston Globe*, 23 January 2020.

1.2

Re-visioning Public Health Ethics
A Relational Perspective

Nuala P. Kenny, Susan B. Sherwin, and Françoise E. Baylis

Canada has a proud tradition of making substantial conceptual advances in public health. With the renewed global interest in public health generated by the H1N1 pandemic, Canada is poised to make significant contributions to the development of a new public health ethics that is firmly grounded in a commitment to the health of populations and communities and to the reduction of health inequalities. However, we are concerned that this opportunity may be squandered by an inordinate focus on issues of emergency-preparedness to the exclusion of the full range of public health concerns[1,2] and an ongoing reliance on bioethical analysis steeped in the individual rights/autonomy discourse of clinical and research ethics.[3-5]

In this paper, we describe some concerns regarding the focus on pandemic ethics in isolation from public health ethics; identify inadequacies in the dominant individualistic ethics framework; and summarize our nascent work on the relational concepts that inform our re-visioning of public health ethics.[6]

Pandemic Ethics: A Narrow Vision
The 2003 Canadian experience of the SARS near-pandemic brought home the reality of fundamental ethical concerns in times of emergency threats to public safety. Among the issues that were identified are restrictions of civil liberties, privacy, the duty of care, the right of health care workers to refuse dangerous work, the right of non-infected patients to access care facilities, the fair distribution of scientific credit for research discoveries, and patent protection.[7,8] While these are important issues, we have argued that,

> [f]rom the perspective of pandemic planning and public health, this is an odd and limited list of concerns—a list that likely would not have been generated but for the fact that the analysis remains steeped in an individual rights discourse inherited from clinical ethics and research ethics, and consonant with the dominant moral and political culture.[6]

Indeed, this analysis situates pandemic as a largely *personal health care issue* when it is in fact a global *public health issue*.

To date, the principle-based approach to ethics generated for clinical care and research, and involving respect for autonomy (of individuals), beneficence, non-maleficence and justice[9] has dominated ethical reflection in all health areas. With this approach, the interests and well-being of individual patients or research subjects are a primary concern. When a health risk affects a population, however, of necessity, the emphasis must shift from individual to collective interests. As the Public Health Agency of Canada recognizes: "When a health risk affects a population,…public health ethics will predominate and a high value will be placed on the collective interests."[10] We join with the Public Health Agency of Canada and others[3,11,12] who call for a social starting point for public health ethics that recognizes community as foundational, and from this perspective caution against pandemic planning in the absence of a robust, population-focused ethic for public health.

At this time, there is no consensus regarding the appropriate theory and method for public health ethics.[2,13,14] It is widely understood, however, that the familiar autonomy-centred principles of contemporary bioethics are clearly inadequate when mapped to the agenda of public health.

Public health ethics requires an approach that is itself "public" rather than individualistic, i.e., one that understands the social nature and goals of public health work. It must make clear the complex ways in which individuals are inseparable from communities and populations and build on the need to attend to the interests of communities and populations as well as individuals.

A Relational Account of Public Health Ethics

We propose an alternative approach to public health ethics that is rooted in a relational understanding of persons. Public health deals with the health needs of communities and populations through actions that are taken at a social and political level. As such, it requires a conception of persons as embedded within communities in particular ways; it should recognize and respond to their fundamental social and political nature, and be attentive to ways in which patterns of systematic discrimination (or privilege) operate in terms of the goals and activities of public health.[15] Where traditional bioethics treats persons as self-contained, self-interested, and self-directing creatures, relational ethics insists that persons be treated as the social, interdependent beings that they are. Relational persons develop and deploy their values within the social worlds they inhabit, conditioned by the opportunities and obstacles that shape their lives according to the socially salient features of their embodied lives (e.g., their gender, race, class, age, disability status, ethnicity).[16]

Relational Autonomy

Autonomy remains an important value because public health involves actions aimed at the common good and the health of populations and it is easy to lose track of the rights and interests of individuals. However, relational autonomy embraces (rather than ignores) the fact that persons are inherently socially, politically, and economically-situated beings. A relational approach to autonomy directs us to attend to the many and varied ways in which competing policy options affect the opportunities available to members of different social groups (for example, quarantine may have a very different impact on those with significant disabilities than it will on those who can look after their own bodily needs), and to make visible the ways in which the autonomy of some may come at the expense of others. Relational autonomy encourages us to see that there are many ways in which autonomy can be compromised. It allows us to see that sometimes autonomy is best promoted through social change rather than simply protecting individuals' freedom to act within existing structures.

Relational Social Justice

The traditional bioethics principle of justice is primarily concerned with non-discrimination and distributive justice (the fair distribution of quantifiable benefits and burdens) among discrete individuals, including allocation of scarce resources such as vaccines or hospital beds. On a relational account, the concern falls more heavily on matters of social justice, involving fair access to social goods such as rights, opportunities, power, and self respect.[17] This view of social justice directs us to explore the context in which certain political and social policies and structures are created and maintained. It asks us to look beyond effects on individuals and to see how members of different social groups may be collectively affected by practices that create inequalities in access and opportunity. Social justice enjoins us to correct *patterns* of systemic injustice among different groups, seeking to improve rather than worsen systematic disadvantages in society. It requires attention to the needs of the most disadvantaged. We join with Powers and Faden in believing that social justice is "the foundational moral justification for public health."[12]

Relational Solidarity

Public health involves efforts to attend to the needs of all, especially the most vulnerable and systematically disadvantaged members of society; as such, it should promote the value of solidarity.[1,7,17] Conventional solidarity refers to common interests, purposes, or sympathies between discrete individuals or among members of a group.[18] Sometimes the emphasis is on altruism and helping relationships, particularly with the needy and disadvantaged. At other times, the emphasis is on reciprocity (with a focus on communality and mutuality) and the benefits of social cohesion. This conventional understanding of solidarity, however, is limited in its usefulness for public health ethics because of its ultimate reliance on the oppositional categories "us" and "them" based on identification with a common cause, a collective identity, and anticipation of mutual advantage among the "us" (usually defined in opposition to some excluded "others"). This understanding of solidarity fails to capture the wider public, many of whom may be among the vulnerable and systematically disadvantaged.

A relational concept of solidarity, built on a relational understanding of personhood and autonomy, aims to expand the category of "us" to "us all" and to do away with the binary opposition at work with the notions of "us" and "them." Relational solidarity values interconnections without being steeped in assumptions about commonality or collective identity in contrast to some other group. What matters in public health is a shared interest in survival, safety and security—an interest that can be effectively pursued through the pursuit of public goods understood as "non-excludable" and "non-rivalrous."[19] There are few pure public goods and health *per se* is not among them. However, there are numerous public goods *for* health, including: scientific knowledge, communicable disease control (including vaccination), and control of antibiotic resistance. Indeed, it is in this function of public health—to promote public goods—that we can best appreciate the role of solidarity at work. In this sense, the meaning of solidarity is found *within* public health itself.

Relational Ethics in the Real World of Public Health Policy

Public health ethics must expand as well as modify the traditional principles of bioethics.

In an earlier paper, we developed an extensive theoretical account of the principles of relational autonomy, relational social justice and relational solidarity,[6] and while there is still much work to be done to further refine these principles, we believe they have an important role to play in the practical and pressured policy world.

Specifically, we believe that these principles can help to reclaim and centre the common and collective good at risk in pandemic and other emergency situations. Indeed, since discussions of common and shared resources are almost impossible to raise in the environment of personal health care, public health may be the only viable source for reflections about our interdependence in times of need.

Minimally, these principles for a relational public health ethic carry with them important procedural and substantive demands. They require a policy-making process that is truly transparent, fair and inclusive, which requires that it be sensitive and responsive to the workings of systemic inequalities. Substantively, these relational principles also require public recognition of the fact that we enter any crisis with varying degrees of inequity and that the public policy response to the crisis must not foreseeably increase existing inequities. These are modest demands but they are easily overlooked within a framework that focuses solely on the rights of individuals apart from their social context.

Public health joins a few other key public goods (e.g., universal education, prevention of further contributions to climate change, avoidance of nuclear war) in helping all to appreciate the reality of our mutual interest in survival, safety and security on the one hand, and our mutual vulnerability to disease, violence and death on the other. Because public health is an essential tool for promoting these very interests, we must come to appreciate the importance of recognizing our common vulnerabilities and needs and see the importance of a commitment to relational public health ethics as the means to achieve the necessary public goods.

References

1 Childress JF, Faden RR, Gaare RD, Gostin LO, Kahn J, Bonnie RJ, et al. Public health ethics: Mapping the terrain. *J Law Med Ethics* 2002;30:170–78.

2 Kass NE. An ethics framework for public health. *Am J Public Health* 2001;91(11):1776–82.

3 Beauchamp DE. Community: The neglected tradition of public health. *Hastings Center Report* 1985;15:28–36.

4 Rogers WA. Feminism and public health ethics. *J Med Ethics* 2008;32:351–54.

5 Jennings B. Public health and civic republicanism: Toward an alternative framework for public health ethics. In: Dawson A, Verweij M (Eds.), *Ethics, Prevention and Public Health.* New York, NY: Oxford University Press, 2007.

6 Baylis F, Kenny NP, Sherwin S. A relational account of public health ethics. *Public Health Ethics* 2008;1(3):196–209.

7 Singer PA, Benatar SR, Bernstein M, Abdallah SD, Dickens BM, MacRae SK, et al. Ethics and SARS: Lessons from Toronto. *BMJ* 2003;327:1342–44.

8 University of Toronto, Joint Centre for Bioethics Pandemic Influenza Working Group. Stand on Guard for Thee: Ethical Considerations in Preparedness Planning for Pandemic Influenza. November 2005 (http://www.jointcentreforbioethics.ca/publications/documents/ stand_on_guard.pdf).

9 Beauchamp TL, Childress JF. *Principles of Biomedical Ethics*, 4th ed. New York: Oxford University Press, 2004.

10 Public Health Agency of Canada. The Canadian Pandemic Influenza Plan for the Health Sector. Section Two: Background. 2006 (http://www.phac-aspc.gc.ca/cpip-pclcpi/pdf-e/ section_2-eng.pdf).

11 Callahan D. Individual good and common good: A communitarian approach to bioethics. *Perspect Biol Med* 2003;46:496–507.

12 Powers M, Faden R. *Social Justice: The Moral Foundations of Public Health and Health Policy.* New York: Oxford University Press, 2006.

13 Roberts MJ, Reich MR. Ethical analysis in public health. *Lancet* 2002;359:1055–59.

14 Upshur RE. Principles for the justification of public health intervention. *Can J Public Health* 2002;93(2):101–03.

15 Sherwin S, and The Canadian Feminist Health Research Network (Eds). A relational approach to autonomy in health care. In: Sherwin S, *The Politics of Women's Health: Exploring Agency and Autonomy.* Philadelphia, PA: Temple University Press, 1998.

16 Young IM. *Justice and the Politics of Difference.* Princeton, NJ: Princeton University Press, 1990.

17 Tauber AI. Medicine, public health and the ethics of rationing. *Perspect Biol Med* 2002; 45:16–30.

18 Houtepen R, ter Muelen R. The expectation(s) of solidarity and identity in the reconstruction of the health care system. *Health Care Analysis* 2006b;8:355–76.

19 Labonté R, Schrecker T. Globalization and social determinants of health: Promoting health equity in global governance (Part 3 of 3). *Globalization and Health* 2007;3, doi:10.1186/1744-8603-3-7 (http://www.globalizationandhealth.com/content/3/1/7).

QUESTIONS FOR REFLECTION

1. Choose a moral issue that arises in pandemics and analyze the issue from the perspective of at least two moral approaches, such as utilitarianism, libertarianism, or relational ethics. How does the use of different moral theories lead to different analyses of the issue? Some issues you might consider:

   a. Does the public have obligations to follow government directives, and if so, when do these obligations arise?

   b. Is it wrong for individuals to hoard items that are needed in a pandemic?

   c. Do businesses have responsibilities to protect their workers, and if so, in what ways?

   d. Do essential businesses, such as grocery stores, have an obligation to offer employees hazard pay?

   e. Do governments have an obligation to subsidize businesses that are financially impacted in a pandemic?

2. How does a relational approach to public health ethics differ from a Rawlsian, utilitarian, libertarian, or communitarian approach? Are there any similarities among all of these different approaches?

2

Professional Responsibilities

INTRODUCTION

Under normal conditions, health-care professionals owe a duty of care to their patients. Does this duty continue to hold when dealing with diseases that are communicable and potentially fatal, such as COVID-19? What are the limits of this duty? Do the obligations entailed by this duty change depending on whether one is a doctor, a nurse, or a personal support worker making minimum wage? Do health-care professionals have a responsibility to treat patients even when they lack personal protective equipment (PPE) and when treatment would require putting themselves and their families at risk?

In the first reading of this section, Udo Schuklenk argues that health-care professionals do not have an obligation to treat in the absence of sufficient PPE. Schuklenk points out that the lack of adequate PPE during the COVID-19 epidemic has resulted directly from cost-cutting measures instituted by Western governments. The fact that these governments have voluntarily chosen to obtain inadequate supplies undermines the moral obligations of health-care workers who have entered their respective professions with the expectation of proper equipment. If health-care professionals continue to treat patients, their actions are morally commendable but not required (they are "supererogatory").

In the next reading, Abbey Lowe, Angela Hewlett, and Toby Schonfeld examine the obligations of health-care professionals toward those in distant parts of the world. They argue that one may have a duty to treat people suffering from outbreaks of highly hazardous communicable diseases, even in other countries and continents. This duty may arise from the moral value of "solidarity" among citizens from different parts of the world, especially given that contagious diseases don't respect national boundaries.

Lastly, Seth Holmes and Liza Buchbinder examine the personal experiences of health-care professionals who have been asked to work in intensive care units without adequate PPE. Many of those people report feeling scared and dreading their upcoming shifts, knowing that they put themselves and others at risk when working without proper equipment. Holmes and Buchbinder point out that shortages of PPE could mean not only that patients and health-care workers are at risk but also that the health-care system itself is at risk of understaffing if those workers fall ill.

KEY TERMS

fiduciary relationship: a relationship in which one party places special trust and confidence in another. This relationship gives rise to fiduciary duties, which include the need to ensure the well-being of the trusting party and act for their benefit. The doctor-patient relationship is a fiduciary relationship that confers fiduciary duties on the doctor.

N95 respirator mask: a mask that fits closely over the face to filter out 95 per cent of particles, including many viruses. The 'N' indicates that the mask is not resistant to oil. The N95 respirator is a standard piece of PPE that has frequently been in short supply during the COVID-19 pandemic.

Public Health Emergency of International Concern (PHEIC): a formal designation from the World Health Organization, defined as "an extraordinary event which is determined, as provided in these Regulations: a) to constitute a public health risk to other States through the international spread of disease; and b) to potentially require a coordinated international response."[1] Before COVID-19 was declared a pandemic, the World Health Organization designated it a PHEIC.

supererogatory: above and beyond what is morally required; doing more than what you are obliged to do. Some have argued that the actions of health-care professionals during the COVID-19 pandemic have been supererogatory.

NOTE

1 World Health Organization (2005), "IHR Procedures Concerning Public Health Emergencies of International Concern (PHEIC)," https://www.who.int/ihr/procedures/pheic/en/.

2.1

Health Care Professionals Are under No Ethical Obligation to Treat COVID-19 Patients

Udo Schuklenk

Even a cursory look at the news tells us that many doctors and nurses are reluctant to provide care to COVID-19 patients. Personal protective equipment (PPE) levels in Australia's state of Queensland are very low, writes the state's Clinical Senate Chair Alex Markwell.[1] Bulgaria has seen a wave of doctors resigning, Zimbabwean doctors have gone on strike over the lack of protective equipment, and UK medics warned repeatedly that the lack of appropriate protective equipment puts their own lives at risk.

These professionals sadly have every reason to be concerned for their own well-being. As of [April 1, 2020], more than 60 doctors who provided care to Italian COVID-19 patients have died as a result of contracting the virus on the job. Many more have fallen very seriously sick. An incomplete list of "Fallen Coronavirus Heroes" maintained by Michael C. Gibson, a Harvard University medical school professor, lists (as of March 31, 2020) 119 health care professionals who lost their lives as a result of COVID-19 infections they acquired while caring for infected patients.

The number is almost certainly significantly higher, and it is bound to increase daily, for some time to come. There can be no doubt, the death toll among health care professionals caring for COVID-19 patients the world all over will be significant. In response to concerns about the availability of health care professionals during expected COVID-19 case surges, a state government in one of Germany's most populous states, North-Rhine Westfalia, is seriously considering introducing a draft kind of compulsory service for health care professionals. Little did doctors know when they joined the profession, that at some point further down the road, government was planning to draft them into compulsory service, much like soldiers.

What Health Care Professionals Owe Us

What is it then that health care professionals owe us in a crisis like the current one? As patients, we depend on doctors and nurses to provide professional care to us, because they have the specialist training, and they have a monopoly on the provision of these kinds of services. It's not as if we could turn around and go elsewhere if the local hospital's ICU has an insufficient number of doctors on call.

Most doctors in their graduation ceremonies do take a public oath to serve the public good, oftentimes modelled on the World Medical Association's Declaration of Geneva. Up to the 1994 version of that influential document doctors promised to provide emergency care, without any ifs or buts. However, you won't find that promise repeated in the current version of that document, so that approach doesn't address the question at hand. Unsurprisingly, the world's doctors woke up to the dangers of making wild promises they could not realistically live up to.

A different argument could be to say that there is an implied consent to risk-taking when doctors accepted the deal their profession cut with society. Monopoly powers, high societal standing and oftentimes high salaries don't come without a price. Doctors knew, if they paid attention to the subject in their global health classes, that infectious agents like Ebola and others were going to raise their ugly heads during their lifetime, and joining the profession meant accepting a duty to provide care. During the early days of the HIV pandemic, when an infection with that virus meant certain death, doctors' statutory bodies declared in most countries that doctors had an obligation to treat. Given COVID-19's much lower mortality risk this should settle it, or so one might think. That is a mistaken view.

What makes COVID-19 different is that the HIV-response was predicated on the availability of PPE to health care professionals. In such a reality, if health care professionals followed universal precautions and had the right protective equipment, the odds of them picking up HIV would have been negligible. With COVID-19 we are, in most countries, in a very different situation.

Yes, We Must Talk about Neoliberalism and the Fetishization of "Efficiency"
One feature closely linked to the functioning of globalisation and capitalism is efficiency. Nobody wants to waste money and resources. There is a virtue in running "lean" operations. Most countries in the global north, that operate public health care systems, saw the re-election of cost-cutting governments running successfully on election campaigns promising to "return money to our back pockets," and away from big government. And as taxpayers we did get money returned to our back pockets by low tax regimes.

As neoliberal election campaign lore has it, we know best how to spend our hard-earned money. Such policies were anything but cost neutral, as those of us in need of public services have known for a long time. They succeeded in hollowing out the health care delivery infrastructures in most countries. There is today not much of a difference between Australia, Germany, Canada and the UK. The principle that drove public policy was the same. In the UK citizens were treated to many years of low-tax, small-state austerity, effectively rendering the NHS unable to cover regular flu season case loads without great difficulty. In Germany the German finance minister's Black Zero signified the fiscal paradigm requiring the state not to run budget deficits, leading equally to a hollowing out of the state infrastructure required to respond efficiently in times not normal. In the USA where publicly funded health care delivery is close to non-existent and for-profit, operators often dictate the levels of care that will be provided. The results were quite similar, except in this case the availability of health care infrastructure was dictated by profit objectives driving many hospitals, as well as for-profit insurers reimbursing for-profit and non-profit hospitals alike for particular services.

Implications for Health Care Professionals' Obligations

The endpoint was the same: democratically elected governments across the global north have left hospitals woefully unprepared for the current onslaught of patients, not only in terms of ICU beds and ventilators, but also in terms of PPE. If the lack of available PPE for frontline health care professionals [had] been due to a natural occurrence, one could argue that doctors should be prepared to accept a certain higher degree of risk, but in the current situation that lack of protective equipment is truly deliberate: it is by human, cost-cutting design. It was quite a remarkable sight to see on global news programmes the UK Chancellor and Prime Minister standing outside 10 Downing Street, wildly applauding the country's health care professionals' heroism. The heroism, however, that they were celebrating is a direct, avoidable consequence of their own government's austerity policies. An adequately resourced NHS would not have required a significant degree of beyond-the-call-of-duty heroism by health care professionals.

We live in democracies, and we elected politicians who promised us that we could have our cake and eat it. It turns out, unsurprisingly, we can't have that. There is no reason why doctors and nurses should be seen to be professionally obliged to risk their well-being today, because we chose governments that starved them of the necessary resources to do their job safely. Elections have consequences.

We should be grateful to any health care professional willing to care for COVID-19 patients, in the absence of PPE, but we have no reason to take for granted that there will be one when we need them.

Note

1 Lydia Lynch, "Queensland hospitals 'very low' on gloves, masks, gowns and told to re-use," *Brisbane Times*, 17 March 2020.

2.2

How Should Clinicians Respond to International Public Health Emergencies?

Abbey Lowe, Angela Hewlett, and Toby Schonfeld

Case

Dr W is a hospital administrator at BB academic medical center in the United States. BB has a prominent global health program, and Dr V, an expert in epidemic responses, has expressed interest in working abroad with Médecins Sans Frontières (MSF—Doctors Without Borders) on the current Ebola outbreak. Upon returning from work in prior Ebola outbreaks, clinicians have been monitored in isolated Ebola units until it can be confirmed that they have not contracted the virus. Despite staff having been "cleared," however, some BB patients worry about attending appointments or coming to a hospital where "some doctors and nurses have been around Ebola." Even some members of BB's staff have stated that they will not treat patients who have a disease as deadly as Ebola out of fear for their own safety. Concerned about bad publicity and media attention, the BB board of directors has asked Dr W to dissuade Dr V from continuing international work on Ebola containment, suggesting that "there are other important global health projects that don't scare people so much." Dr W wonders how to respond.

Commentary

Health care workers (HCWs) are holders of privileged knowledge and of the public's trust; they have a sacred duty in society—that of healers. In return for the public's trust, they owe a duty to care based on their fiduciary relationship to patients.[1] In the legal sense, the phrase *a duty of care* stems from a special relationship between a physician and his or her patient—a relationship that is voluntary and entered into by mutual agreement.[2] Certainly, this definition is clear when applied to a cardiologist treating a patient presenting at the hospital with chest pain. However, what is the obligation of an expert in epidemic responses, like Dr V, to those suffering from highly hazardous communicable diseases in the midst of an epidemic?

There is little consensus on the extent to which health care workers have a duty to provide health services in an outbreak or what that duty might entail.[3] Explicating the duty to care in a public health emergency of international concern (PHEIC) comes with hurdles. The challenges stemming from a PHEIC might include: (1) difficulty in defining hospitals' obligations to multiple groups—employees, patients, and the community; (2) providing safe working conditions for HCWs; (3) operating in a health care system with different standards of care; and (4) providing compensation and time off for HCWs to travel to impacted areas.[1]

Without clear formulation of the duty to care in a PHEIC, HCWs as well as academic medical center leadership may end up overwhelmed by the challenges of serving in an outbreak-afflicted area. Yakubu et al. assert that there is not a professional duty to treat in these circumstances, only a moral one.[4] Yet here we will argue that, given the landscape of outbreaks of international concern, Dr V's expressed interest and altruism in serving abroad are not merely issues of personal conscience; they exemplify the value of solidarity that institutions like BB academic medical center and society should encourage.[5]

Global Health Solidarity
British bioethicists Prainsack and Buyx define solidarity as an "enacted commitment to carry 'costs' (financial, social, emotional, or otherwise) to assist others with whom a person or persons recognize similarity in a relevant respect."[6] Our shared vulnerability to highly hazardous communicable diseases (HHCDs)— diseases that only know the boundaries of biology and don't respect national borders—should incite a shared responsibility to fight an HHCD outbreak together.[7] The similarity that exists between a patient at BB academic medical center and an individual living in the Democratic Republic of the Congo (DRC) is that both are increasingly united in their vulnerability to emerging threats. Consider a US citizen returning from a visit to the DRC on a full plane back to the US sitting in seat 52B. Two days later, a passenger who had been seated in 52A begins to feel nauseous. Ten days after returning to his home, the passenger who had been seated in 52C visits the emergency room with a high fever and vomiting. Even with safeguards, exposure can build exponentially. An outbreak in the DRC, if not contained, will spread to countries on different continents, just as it has spread to countries within Africa. Although the United States and Europe have been successful in treating patients with known Ebola virus disease (EVD) through airlifting them and treating them in specialized biocontainment units, these are limited resources.[7] If exposures and known cases breach the limits of those resources, controlling the spread of EVD is likely to tax the US health care system and threaten the health security of the US population. The duty to care for those suffering on the other side of the globe may be strengthened by greater recognition of our shared vulnerability and a commitment to solidarity toward a shared threat. Solidaristic practices would entail taking action to care for those suffering abroad with the support of the government and institutions, just as if the outbreak were on US soil.[8]

Dr V's desire to serve in an area affected by the outbreak, putting her life at risk, demonstrates solidarity—to be in solidarity with others is to act on their behalf and to accept the costs of doing so.[8] However, her risk is not hers alone. Dr V's actions stand to affect BB's patients as well as the community at large. As such, BB academic medical center's board of directors is correctly concerned about the risk of exposure to current patients and assuaging fear of community members, who, along with BB patients and some staff, might perceive the ongoing work done by BB medical center's participating staff as a threat to their safety. BB patients and staff may be especially concerned about being exposed to Ebola by BB clinicians returning from working in the outbreak-affected area.

Health care institutions should have a strategy for managing the risk of exposure to patients and employees from returning staff who have worked in outbreak-afflicted areas, as it is possible to manage the risk of this exposure effectively. Clinical staff should be required to register their travel and prospectively commit to complying with Centers for Disease Control and Prevention guidelines for managing potential Ebola virus exposure[9] on their return, as these guidelines have proven effective in US monitoring of health care professionals returning from EVD outbreak environments.[10] With these controls in place, physical risks are manageable; they should not dominate the discourse about supporting international service.

Supporting HCWs' service in a PHEIC through organizations like MSF contributes to their safety and mitigates their risk of contracting disease. However, an additional concern for BB's board of directors is that the BB patient community feel adequately safeguarded; BB academic medical center upholds its reputation as a trusted institution in the community. Dr W should respond to BB's board of directors by providing a clear explanation of the physical risks to HCWs working with MSF and the likelihood of their contracting an HHCD. In addition, Dr W should detail a plan to mitigate the risk of exposure to patients along with a communication strategy designed to provide transparent responses to patients' concerns and to garner trust within the BB community.

Solidarity is often an implicit prerequisite among groups for the delivery and maintenance of important social infrastructures.[7] Public health programs such as vaccination campaigns or routine water sampling—or infrastructure like the justice system—work on behalf of the public and are funded through the government. Solidarity could underlie the approach to global health threats, as academic medical centers with prominent global health programs, such as BB, could commit a portion of their funds to strengthening health care infrastructure in affected countries. If BB academic medical center's board of directors see the community as vulnerable to the threat of HHCDs, supporting a range of efforts to contain a disease might be easier to "sell" to their patients and community. BB academic medical center and hospitals who mobilize qualified HCWs to work in affected areas could not only meet the needs of desperate patients but also contain Ebola at its source, averting global risk.

Solidarity in Practice

Pursuing global health solidarity could be an aspirational component of a global health program's mission, but implementing it is not without difficulty for academic medical centers. Supporting health care workers who go abroad to assist in mitigating an outbreak takes careful consideration on the part of academic medical centers concerning the risks employees may face—ranging from contracting HHCDs to potentially working amidst political instability and violence. For academic medical centers with global health programs, steps should be taken to ensure that staff members in the field are adequately supported and that the institution has staffing coverage, especially when sending a team of health care workers for an extended period of time.

Local support. Uncertainty surrounds the continued availability of medical evacuation for staff, and there may also be concerns regarding violence and civil unrest in Ebola-affected countries.[11] Dr V cannot be expected to shoulder this risk alone but rather should receive support from BB academic medical center, which might worry about whether it can adequately protect its employees. To minimize the risks and maximize the benefits of HCWs' service, academic medical centers and other institutions should require that HCWs who volunteer to serve do so only through established and qualified organizations and should help HCWs to inform themselves fully of all residual risks and uncertainties.[5]

Staffing coverage. BB academic medical center's commitment to support HCWs serving in an outbreak-afflicted area also requires consideration of the strain it will place on its staff and patients. Providing care in Ebola-affected regions can involve an extensive time commitment for clinicians—not only time spent deployed but also several days of training and sometimes several weeks postdeployment away from work for monitoring, if required.[5] On the clinical side, Dr V's time away from work could increase BB clinicians' patient load, create strain on colleagues who are tasked with covering extra responsibilities, and jeopardize continuity of physician care. Although it will be necessary for academic medical centers to address these concerns, the number of HCWs willing and qualified to serve is small, and the strain on institutions and staff members is likely to be minor.[5]

Conclusion

In an editorial in the Bulletin of the World Health Organization, Flahault et al. argue that respect for human rights and solidarity should be at the heart of each country's national security agenda; furthermore, the authors claim that these values are consistent with the motives of many people who provide health services in public health emergencies.[12] BB academic medical center and its leadership should consider how solidarity fits with the mission of the institution's global health program. Solidarity practices should be communicated to and reinforced within the institution and community. Such efforts can make inroads in garnering support from BB staff, patients, and community stakeholders in supporting HCWs willing to act on their sense of solidarity.

References

1 Thompson A. Bioethics meets Ebola: exploring the moral landscape. *Br Med Bull.* 2016; 117(1):5–13.

2 Shensky ES. What is a healthcare provider's duty to care? *National Law Review.* October 19, 2015. https://www.natlawreview.com/article/what-healthcare-provider-s-duty-care. Accessed on July 9, 2019.

3 Ruderman C, Tracy CS, Bensimon CM, et al. On pandemics and the duty to care: whose duty? Who cares? *BMC Med Ethics.* 2006;7:e5.

4 Yakubu A, Folayan MO, Sani-Gwarzo N, et al. The Ebola outbreak in Western Africa: ethical obligations for care. *J Med Ethics.* 2016;42(4):209–210.

5 Mello M, Merritt M, Halpern S. Supporting those who go to fight Ebola. *PLoS Med.* 2015;12(1):e1001781.

6 Prainsack B, Buyx A. *Solidarity: Reflections on an Emerging Concept in Bioethics.* London, UK: Nuffield Council on Bioethics; 2011.

7 West-Oram PGN, Buyx A. Global health solidarity. *Public Health Ethics.* 2017;10(2):212–224.

8 Uyeki TM, Mehta AK, Davey RT Jr, et al; Working Group of the US-European Clinical Network on Clinical Management of Ebola Virus Disease Patients in the US and Europe. Clinical management of Ebola virus disease in the United States and Europe. *New Engl J Med.* 2016;374(7):636–646.

9 Centers for Disease Control and Prevention. Interim US guidance for monitoring and movement of persons with potential Ebola virus exposure. https://www.nalc.org/workplace-issues/body/2014-10-29-CDC-Update-on-monitoring-and-movement-of-persons-with-Potential-Ebola.pdf. Updated November 28, 2014. Accessed May 28, 2019.

10 Stehling-Ariza T, Fisher E, Vagi S, et al. Monitoring of persons with risk for exposure to Ebola virus disease—United States, November 3, 2014–March 8, 2015. *MMWR Morb Mortal Wkly Rep.* 2015;64(25):685–689.

11 Mangan K. Universities curtail health experts' efforts to work on Ebola in West Africa. *Chron High Educ.* 2014;61(9):A12.

12 Flahault A, Didier W, Zylberman P, et al. From global health security to global health solidarity, security and sustainability. *Bull World Health Organ.* 2016;94(12):863.

2.3

In a Defunded Health System, Doctors and Nurses Suffer Near-Impossible Conditions

Seth Holmes and Liza Buchbinder

"This virus is deadly, but they're throwing us into the fire and saying, 'oh well.'"

The doctor who said this continues to show up daily, caring for patients in need. Her health—and that of millions of other doctors, nurses, their families and the patients they care for—is put at risk when our leaders de-fund the health system that protects us all. She and other front line health workers, covering extra shifts and working overtime in this historic pandemic, tap into reserves of strength and resilience in hopes that the long overdue staff, equipment, space and systems arrive before the cases of COVID-19 surge out of control.

One Seattle area critical care physician, working in the intensive care unit (ICU) told us this past week, "I'm trying not to get too freaked out, but it's hard." Another called us from a large, urban hospital on the West Coast said, "It's very scary and I've panicked many times. But what can you do?"

Another nurse from a rural hospital told us: "I'm going in to work in the hospital tonight. There's a patient positive for COVID-19 in the ICU. Dreading to go in, but obviously wouldn't call out of my shifts."

These are the distressed voices of our friends and colleagues—frontline health workers entering hospitals every day, working overtime, covering extra shifts in this historic pandemic. Our friends, colleagues and co-workers have asked not to be named for fear of losing their jobs in this uncertain time.

We are acutely aware of how contagious and deadly the virus is—especially for elderly and chronically ill people. Yet, we and our patients are put at unnecessary risk due to shortages of basic protective health equipment and testing kits. These shortages were avoidable and they never should have happened. The Trump administration's active de-funding of our health system is leading to additional exposures, infections and deaths.

We have trained over many years to calmly soldier on in the face of the turmoil, suffering and pain that plays out every day in health care. But the avoidable shortages of basic equipment in this pandemic add layers of uncertainty and strain that are pushing providers and our health system toward the breaking point.

THE ETHICS OF PANDEMICS

Another colleague and single mother of two young girls shared this week, "All these other moms are sharing color coded schedules to keep kids busy and I'm thinking I just don't want to end up in the ICU as a COVID statistic." A nurse working in a large, private hospital in a major US city explained, "Our hospital alone has had close to 300 cases. The latest person to test positive has been in the hospital for over 90 days. Who knows how many of us have been exposed?"

Yet, what causes fear most for front line physicians and nurses is not the COVID-19 virus itself nor even the Severe Acute Respiratory Syndrome it can cause, but rather the lack of protective equipment and testing kits. The lack of protective equipment—including N95 masks—and the lack of test kits to diagnose and treat patients make it nearly impossible for us to care effectively for patients. Without this basic protection, dozens of clinicians in the US have already contracted COVID-19.[1] Others are on mandatory home quarantine, unable to work as they wait to know their own fates. Some are currently intubated on ventilators in ICUs as patients themselves. Many continue to work in the midst of fear and uncertainty. And many more are on mandatory standby for COVID deployment—what could become effectively a medical draft.

Echoing statements from other friends and colleagues across the country, a nurse in New York City shared, "I don't think hospital staff should be destined to contract COVID just because there's a lack of Personal Protective Equipment. I did not sign up to die because of a lack of PPE!"

A physician in an outpatient clinic in the Midwest explained, "Clinic gets hairier every week. Still can't believe we can't do testing." Another physician in a hospital in the South stated, "This is not that hard—get us what we need so we can work. We will work, just with the right equipment. How is this even a roadblock in a country like the US?"

Due to avoidable shortages, many hospitals now require doctors and nurses to re-use masks day after day, sometimes for more than 30 days—prompting the Twitter hashtag #GiveMePPE. The lack of equipment also leads to policies prohibiting clinicians from using protective masks even when concerned for our own safety, unless caring directly for a patient designated a "Person Under Investigation." Due to lack of simple synthetic nasal swabs, we are prohibited from ordering tests for many patients in whom we suspect COVID-19—even if the patients have a fever or cough and predisposing condition. These policies are not due to rational, evidence-based medicine. Rather, they stem from a lack of "staff, stuff, space and systems."[2]

In the words of one of our physician co-workers this week, "Unless hospitals want to burn through their doctors and nurses with us all in quarantine, they better let us protect ourselves." A medical school classmate of ours now working in a level one trauma center added: "I'm not going into another room with a patient being ruled out for COVID-19 without an N95 mask. Period. They can fire me and the rest of the doctors and nurses who feel similarly."

The lack of basic equipment is not due to the pandemic itself. Rather, the effects of the virus are intensified by the active de-funding of our health system by the Trump administration.

Since his inauguration, Trump has left almost half our scientific leadership positions unfilled.[3] In 2018, the CDC was forced to close or downsize its efforts to fight global epidemic outbreaks in 39 of 40 countries, including China. That same year, the Trump administration dismantled the National Security Council's global health security unit and recalled $252 million of emergency funds for rapid response to outbreaks.[4] In 2019, the Trump administration closed the US Agency for International Development's program working with researchers across the world to respond to viruses. And Trump's 2021 budget released [in February 2020] includes $3 billion in further cuts to core federal agencies including global health response programs. As Robert Reich, former Secretary of Labor, pointed out, in many senses we do not have a public health system. Instead, we work in a for-profit healthcare system that is disjointed and ill-prepared for this and future crises.[5]

We are not sure how long this can continue—especially as more health professionals are quarantined or become sick themselves. Instead, we must stand with frontline health workers and their patients, demanding health and social systems that serve all people, fully funded and supported with staff, stuff, space and systems.

The cuts to the health system are adding fuel to a fire that is now burning out of control. As a society, we must begin to see health and social systems, as well as the frontline doctors and nurses working within them, as more important than the banks and corporations we rush to bail out. In this moment, our lives are in their hands.

Notes

1 Lenny Bernstein, Shawn Boburg, Maria Sacchetti, and Emma Brown, "COVID-19 hits doctors, nurses and EMTs, threatening health system," *Washington Post*, 17 March 2020.

2 Bob Herman, "Paul Farmer on the coronavirus: 'This is another caregivers' disease,'" *Axios*, 9 March 2020.

3 Anita Desikan, "The Trump Administration Has Hindered Our Ability to Effectively Respond to the Coronavirus Epidemic," *Union of Concerned Scientists*, 27 February 2020.

4 Kiera Butler, "Let Us Count the Ways the Trump Administration Is Underprepared to Tackle the Coronavirus," *Mother Jones*, 30 January 2020; "Statement from AFT on Departure of Rear Adm. Timothy Ziemer," *American Federation of Teachers*, 11 May 2018.

5 Robert Reich, "Coronavirus Is Revealing a Secret—America Has No Real Public Health System," *Newsweek*, 17 March 2020.

CASE STUDY

Health Care without PPE

Natalie Argento works as a certified nursing assistant[1] in a long-term care facility. Her husband Todd is a trucker and is often away from home for long stretches. They have two small boys, aged three and five, and they also live with Todd's elderly parents.

Typically, Natalie's responsibilities at the facility include toileting, dressing, and bathing residents—some of the more overlooked duties that are nonetheless vital to the proper functioning of a long-term care facility. Natalie's home life limits her to part-time work, but when Todd isn't driving she sometimes takes full-time nightshifts, during which she cleans rooms and preps meals. Always, her job requires assessing residents' needs and calling in a registered or licensed practical nurse when necessary.

Natalie knows that the facility is perpetually understaffed. There are 130 residents, but sometimes as few as three CNAs on shift at night. On her day shifts Natalie is responsible for 16 residents, about double the number that she believes to be optimal; this amounts to a mere half-hour per resident, per shift. Giving a single bath to a resident sometimes takes that long.

When COVID-19 arrived, the already short-staffed facility went downhill fast. Less than a week after the first resident tested positive, residents and staff throughout the facility developed symptoms. Many staff members stayed home, either quarantined after positive tests or too afraid to come in. Adequate personal protective equipment (PPE) was scarce, if available at all, and staff were forced to re-use non-standard disposable masks.

When Natalie went in for the first time after the outbreak, a chilling scene greeted her. Where normally 20 CNAs and a dozen nurses might be on shift, now Natalie had trouble finding anyone at all. She eventually located the receptionist, Lanelle, who was in a resident's room assisting with bathing care that was well outside of her job description. Lanelle was visibly exhausted, and she told Natalie that only three nurses were on duty and perhaps three more CNAs.

Natalie was met by death in the very next room she visited. The resident had evidently passed away overnight. He had been bedridden, and was lying in sheets stained up to his shoulders with excrement. No one had changed his diapers in days. Natalie could barely breathe. The conditions everywhere were grisly. Other patients were drenched in urine, dehydrated, unfed, confused, or panicked. Some, unable to move by themselves, could only lie in bed and pray for someone to come.

No "hot zone" for infected patients had been established, and some residents, known to be infected, were wandering around the floor. Natalie proceeded to work 16 hours without a break, and when she eventually left to return home she did so knowing that most residents were still dehydrated, hungry, and unchanged.

Though scheduled to return the next day, Natalie stayed home. She felt that the risk of infecting herself and spreading infection to her family, co-workers, and others was too great. She also assumed that emergency staff would be on the way and better equipped to protect themselves from infection.

Over the next two days, she received numerous phone calls from the facility. She answered the first of these calls and explained her unwillingness to work, but the calls continued. The scheduler pleaded over voicemail, arguing that Natalie's knowledge of the home was essential, that her co-workers needed her, and that the residents relied on her—they were dying by the day, three and four at a time. How could Natalie with good conscience stay away?

Natalie had trouble sleeping. She had of course chosen freely to enter the profession, and to her understanding she had no legal obligation to continue working at the facility if she declined her proposed shifts and clearly expressed her unwillingness to continue in the absence of suitable PPE. But she knew that her specialized training and familiarity with the facility put her in a unique position—not just anyone could substitute in and help the residents in the way that she could.

Does Natalie's professional expertise entail moral obligations to continue delivering care, even if she has no such legal obligations? If so, how should Natalie weigh those obligations to the facility's residents against her own safety concerns?

PPE at the facility is scarce, and to continue delivering care in the hazardous environment of the virus-riddled hospital would mean acting against the instructions Natalie received in her formal job training. To what degree do Natalie's obligations depend on her access to effective PPE? Should she bend the rules in light of the unusual circumstance of the pandemic and the distress of the residents? If the facility's management team had done everything in its power to attain suitable PPE but had been unable to provide the equipment due to national or global shortages, would this have any bearing on whether Natalie should continue working?

Would Natalie's obligations differ if instead she was a registered nurse or doctor? Why?

Note

1   A Certified Nursing Assistant (CNA) program in the United States typically takes four to eight weeks to complete and is state-certified. Programs in Canada for equivalent positions (Personal Support Worker, Health Care Aid, Patient Attendant) take anywhere from 6 to 12 months to complete but are not certified.

QUESTIONS FOR REFLECTION

1. Do health-care professionals have an obligation to treat patients during outbreaks of highly hazardous communicable diseases? Do the same obligations hold for all health-care professionals, including physicians, nurses, technicians, medical administrative staff, etc.?

2. If health-care professionals do have an obligation to treat patients during outbreaks, are there any limits to these obligations? Are the obligations diminished if inadequate PPE is available?

3. Do citizens have obligations toward health-care professionals who put themselves at risk to treat them during outbreaks of highly hazardous communicable diseases? If so, what are these obligations and what are their limits?

4. Do essential workers in other industries such as food production and delivery services have obligations to continue working in the context of a pandemic or other health-care emergency? If so, how do these obligations arise? Unlike health-care professionals, it's not normally thought that grocery-store clerks and couriers owe a duty of care. Is there some other duty that they owe to customers or to society at large?

3

Public Adherence

INTRODUCTION

One of the first and most significant measures instituted to contain COVID-19 was the recommendation that people stay away from each other. The terms used for this have varied and shifted over the course of the pandemic. We were first told to practice "social distancing," but then it was decided that we should remain in social solidarity even as we remained physically apart, so the term shifted to "physical distancing." It has at times been difficult to understand precisely what is required. In some contexts, public health authorities have invoked terms common in public health parlance without clearly explaining what they mean in practice. In others, the official advice has changed rapidly from one day to the next or has differed depending on which authority you trust (not all politicians have provided advice consistent with that of public health experts). When public health messaging is confusing, it is not only more difficult for people to follow the instructions of authorities but also more likely that they will express doubt about the reliability of those instructions. At the same time, public adherence may be the single most effective measure in reducing the harm caused by a pandemic illness.

The public health measures instituted in response to COVID-19 are not new. The practice of isolating the sick and tracing their contacts dates back to the bubonic plague outbreaks in late-medieval and early-modern Europe.[1] When Paul Revere received a presidential appointment to the Board of Health in 1799, Boston experienced an outbreak of yellow fever. To control the spread, 1,820 individuals were placed in quarantine on Rainsford Island.[2] In the context of COVID-19, different countries have taken different approaches to enforcing public health directives. Some have employed strict and rigorous measures, as in China's eastern province of Jiangsu, where authorities have used metal poles to barricade apartments, making it easier to monitor people's arrivals and departures.[3] Philippine President Rodrigo Duterte threatened his citizens: "My orders to the police and military...if there is trouble and there's an occasion that they fight back and your lives are in danger, shoot them dead."[4] Other countries have opted for lax enforcement, not even issuing fines for protests that violate prohibitions on large gatherings.[5] No matter the level of enforcement, no country has the capacity to monitor all of its citizens all of the time, so public acceptance of pandemic-related restrictions and advice is essential. There are prudential reasons that people should adhere to public health guidelines, but are there moral requirements to do so?

This chapter opens with a reading by Tom Douglas, who argues that there are moral obligations to follow quarantine orders. Douglas notes that quarantine is often thought of as a blameless punishment because most people subject to it have done nothing wrong in coming into contact with SARS-CoV-2. But does it really amount to punishment of the innocent? Quarantine begins with a reasonable state demand that individuals stay at home. Only those failing to comply with that demand will be subject to state force. And so, Douglas argues, those who break quarantine have committed a moral wrong by putting the lives of others at risk.

In the next reading, Charles M. Blow observes that it is more difficult for some groups to comply with physical distancing measures than it is for others. The working poor, including many African American and Hispanic people, are unlikely to be able to work from home, so they are forced to be in contact with other people or risk unemployment. Blow argues that social distancing is a privilege: those who are able to work from home for a sustained period should be mindful of the fact that not everyone is in the same situation and should take this into account before scolding others.

KEY TERMS

isolation: in the context of COVID-19, the practice of isolation is that of separating those who are infected from those who are not.

physical (social) distancing: a social practice in which healthy individuals are asked to stay home and leave only for essential reasons (e.g., for one member of the household to buy groceries once a week or to perform essential work). When leaving the home, physical distancing policies typically advise that one stay at least 6 feet (2 meters) away from others. The purpose behind these policies is to reduce the number of opportunities for a person to unintentionally spread illness to others. This is especially important for diseases such as COVID-19, where a contagious carrier of the virus may fail to exhibit symptoms and so may not know that they are infected. Physical distancing differs from isolation and quarantine in that it is applied to everyone in a population, including healthy individuals who have not been exposed to the virus.

quarantine: a practice in which those who have may have been exposed are separated from others for a period of time. Quarantine measures may be required in a number of different circumstances, such as when a person returns from travel in a region where infection rates are high.

self-isolation: a heightened practice of physical distancing in which individuals who exhibit symptoms, who are ill, or who are particularly vulnerable to infection or illness are asked to stay home and only leave in the event of emergency (such as for an urgent trip to a medical facility). This is sometimes called voluntary quarantine.

shelter in place: an official order issued during an emergency directing individuals to find a safe location indoors and stay there until they are given an "all clear" or told to evacuate. Shelter in place orders have been used by some jurisdictions during the COVID-19 pandemic. They are also used in response to other emergencies, such as active shooters, tornados, or the release of hazardous materials.

NOTES

1 Paul Slack (1988), "Responses to Plague in Early Modern Europe: The Implications of Public Health," *Social Research* 55(3): 433–53.
2 Nina Rodwin (9 April 2020), "Preventing the Virus 'which walketh in darkness': Rainsford Island, Paul Revere and the Board of Health," *The Paul Revere House*, https://www.paulreverehouse.org/preventing-the-virus-which-walketh-in-darkness-rainsford-island-paul-revere-and-the-board-of-health/.
3 Paul Mozur (3 February 2020), "China, Desperate to Stop Coronavirus, Turns Neighbor against Neighbor," *New York Times*.
4 Martin Petty (1 April 2020), "'Shoot them dead'—Philippine Leader Says Won't Tolerate Lockdown Violators," *Reuters*.
5 Marc Montgomery (18 May 2020), "Toronto Sees Largest Anti-Lockdown Protest so Far," *Radio Canada International*.

3.1

Flouting Quarantine

Tom Douglas[1]

As I write this [on March 24, 2020], COVID-19, an illness caused by the new coronavirus SARS-CoV-2, is sweeping the globe. Over 15,000 people have died, and it is likely that at least one hundred times this many have been infected with the virus.[2]

The outbreak has brought the ethics of quarantine, isolation and enforced social distancing to public attention. Singapore, Hong Kong, Taiwan, South Korea and China have been praised in the press for their rigorous deployment of quarantine and other liberty-restricting measures. By contrast, the US and UK have been widely criticised for their relatively lax approach.

There are differences between quarantine (which applies to individuals who may have been exposed to an infection), isolation (which applies to individuals who are ill) and enforced social distancing (which largely preserves freedom of movement), but for the purposes of this post, I'll treat all three together under the heading of "quarantine." I'll use this term loosely to refer to all interventions that significantly constrain a person's freedom of movement and/or association in order to lower the risk that the person will infect others.

Quarantine, thus understood, restricts the freedom of some individuals—those who are quarantined—in order to reduce the threat that they pose to others.[3] In this respect, it is similar to some defensive measures employed in war (think: imprisoning enemy combatants) and the detention of criminal offenders for the purpose of public protection (think: refusing parole on the basis that an offender remains too dangerous). But the ethical rationales given for quarantine are in one important respect different from the rationales given for these other defensive measures.

Defensive measures deployed in the context of war or criminal justice are often thought to be justified in part on the basis that the individuals who pose a threat to others have committed some wrong that is closely connected to threat.[4] Perhaps, for example, they have come to pose a threat as a result of their own wrongdoing. By contrast, quarantine is usually thought to be justified on grounds that are insensitive to wrongdoing. That is to say, the justifications given for quarantine do not typically make any reference to wrongdoing on the part of the quarantined individuals, or to any factor (such as culpability) that would depend on their wrongdoing.[5]

"Many think of health policy as a realm in which judgments about wrong-doing have no place."

This difference is most easily seen in discussions of proportionality. Defensive measures—whether in war, criminal justice, or infectious disease control—are often thought to be subject to a proportionality constraint: the defensive measure may be employed only if it is proportionate. To what must it be proportionate? In war and criminal justice, the answer is often that it must be proportionate to the gravity of the wrong that has been committed by the individual(s) who will now be targeted by the defensive measure.[6] By contrast, in infectious disease control, the claim is typically that defensive measures must be proportionate to the public health benefit that they can be expected to produce.[7] Wrongdoing is irrelevant.

At first glance, I suspect that this difference will seem natural to many. Many think of health policy as a realm in which judgments about wrongdoing have no place. This can be seen in the widespread acceptance of the view that patients are entitled to necessary medical treatments regardless of whether they wrongfully caused their own illnesses, or of whether treating the illness can be expected to result in their committing a serious crime.

It may also seem that, if they are to succeed, justifications for quarantine will *have* to be insensitive to wrongdoing, for the simple reason that most quarantined individuals will not have committed any wrong in connection to the threat they now pose. Most people with infectious diseases became infected in ways that they either could not have been expected to foresee, or could not have been expected to avoid.

On reflection, though, I wonder whether wrongdoing may have a greater role to play in justifying quarantine than is often thought.

In some cases, people surely *did* acquire their infectious disease through some kind of wrongdoing. They may, for example, have acquired the disease through reckless sexual practices, or unjustifiably refusing to have themselves vaccinated. In other cases, people may *continue* to exhibit a disease as a result of some wrong, such as a wrongful refusal to employ safe and effective treatments which they have been offered.

Of course, most quarantine measures—including those being deployed against COVID-19 currently—are not targeted at individuals who have committed either of these sorts of wrongs. Still, I think wrongdoing might be relevant to their justification.

To see why, note that quarantine doesn't normally involve immediately rounding people up and forcibly moving them into a quarantine facility. Often it instead begins with a state *demand*, with state force entering the scene only when individuals fail to comply with that demand. We can thus distinguish between two elements of quarantine: what we might call "self-quarantine demands" and subsequent "quarantine enforcement."

In the course of the current crisis, for instance, many governments have demanded of some people who may be infected that they stay within their homes for a certain period of time. (As I write this, my own family is halfway through a 14-day period of voluntary self-isolation.) *Some* states have taken further measure of using force against those who fail to comply with those demands.[8] ...

So suppose that a state makes a self-quarantine demand. Perhaps it requires people who develop a cough and live in an area with a high prevalence of COVID-19 to remain in their homes for seven days. Suppose also that this demand is reasonable. But suppose that some people—quarantine-breakers—do not comply with the demand, and are subject to state enforcement: the police forcibly return them to their homes.

In this sort of scenario, all individuals actually subjected to state force—i.e., quarantine enforcement—will be individuals who have previously failed to comply with a self-quarantine demand. In most cases, breaking the quarantine in this way will be morally wrong—in part because it risks the health of others, and in part because it involves a failure to comply with the reasonable demand of a legitimate government. This, it seems to me, might be relevant to the justification of quarantine enforcement. For instance, it is plausible that in wrongfully flouting a self-quarantine demand, one makes oneself *liable* to forms of state intrusion that would otherwise be unjustified.

What difference might this make in the real world?

First, it might bear on *who* may or should be quarantined. It will generally be impractical (and undesirable) for public health authorities to make fine-grained assessments of the wrongs committed by individual quarantine-breakers. Such assessments might have to examine, for example, whether a person is flouting the demand because they don't care about infecting other people, or because they don't understand that the demand is reasonable (perhaps because they have been fed false information about the disease in question). This would clearly be unworkable. Quarantine measures have to be implemented at a population level, and on the basis of simple and easy-to-apply criteria.

But there may be certain broad generalisations that can reasonably be made by those responsible for implementing quarantine. For example, it is plausible to think that adults who flout quarantine demands will generally have committed more serious wrongs than children who flout them, since adults will typically have both a better understanding of the demands, and more control over their compliance with them. It is also plausible to think that those with "office jobs" that can easily be done from home commit more serious wrongs in breaking "stay at home" quarantine than, for example, do workers on zero-hour contracts in the service sector, given the large difference in the costs of observing quarantine for these two groups. An upshot may be that quarantine enforcement will be especially hard to justify when many of those subject to it are children, and relatively easier to justify when many subject to it are office workers.

> "it is plausible that in wrongfully flouting a self-quarantine demand, one makes oneself *liable* to forms of state intrusion that would otherwise be unjustified."

Second—and I think more important—the wrongdoing of many quarantine-breakers may make quarantine enforcement easier to justify than many in the public health community (and, for that matter, the current British government) have assumed. Discussions of quarantine have tended to proceed on the basis that quarantine involves inflicting burdens on innocent individuals, and in part for this reason it has been assumed that quarantine is justified only in extreme circumstances—the justificatory bar is very high. But if the thoughts I offer above are sound, some types of quarantine—those that merely enforce reasonable self-quarantine demands—are in fact imposed on individuals who have typically committed a wrong. This, I think, will lower the justificatory bar, widening the range of cases in which it is permissible for states to enforce quarantine and, indeed, the range of cases in which it is obligatory for them to enforce it.

Whether this will make a difference to the moral status of particular quarantine measures now being implemented, or considered, in relation to COVID-19 will depend, though, on what is morally constraining the use of these measures. A number of different factors have been cited as constraints: that the measures might be unsustainable, and thus counterproductive in the long term; that they might have too-great economic costs; and that they might infringe upon the rights of individuals. Only the last of these constraints would be loosened by the wrongdoing of quarantine-breakers.

Notes

1 I thank Gabriel De Marco, Katrien Devolder and Romy Eskens for comments on a draft of this post.
2 It is thought that the virus has around a 1% mortality rate, suggesting that the circa 15,000 deaths caused to date are the result of around 150,000 infections around four weeks ago (there is a time lag of around four weeks from infection to death). Infection is currently increasing rapidly, so we can expect that many more individuals will have been infected since that time.
3 I mean here that quarantine foreseeably harms the quarantined individuals in *some respect*, not that it harms them overall.
4 There are complications regarding precisely how we understand wrongdoing. Acting in a way that is, all things considered, impermissible? Infringing the rights of another? Infringing the rights of another without sufficient justification? There are also questions about whether the wrongdoing has to be *responsible* or *culpable* or could be *blameless*. Unfortunately I can't get into these complications here.

5 This difference has not eluded theorists of criminal justice. Indeed, the insensitivity of justifications of quarantine to wrongdoing, and thus to moral responsibility for wrongdoing,
   has made quarantine seem an attractive model for moral responsibility sceptics who nevertheless wish to preserve something akin to contemporary criminal justice practices. Gregg
   Caruso and Derek Pereboom have both developed the idea that, even if we are never morally
   responsible for anything, something akin to prevailing criminal justice practices might be
   justified on the same basis that quarantine is justified.

6 See, for example, the first chapter of [*Punishment and Responsibility: Essays in the Philosophy
   of Law*] by H.L.A. Hart. In what follows, I assume that the gravity of a wrong will depend on
   both the strength of the moral obligations violated by the wrongdoer and their culpability
   for violating them. Some might prefer to understand the gravity of a wrong in a way that is
   independent of culpability.

7 See, for example, p. 173 of ["Public Health Ethics: Mapping the Terrain" (James F. Childress,
   et al.), *The Journal of Law, Medicine, & Ethics*, vol. 3, no. 2, 24 January 2007].

8 [For two examples, see Sam Sherwood, "Coronavirus: Tourists to Be Deported from NZ
   for Having No Plans to Self-Isolate," *Stuff*, 17 March 2020; David Boroff, "LOCK HIM UP:
   Coronavirus Patient under 24/7 Armed Guard after REFUSING to Self-Isolate," *The US Sun*,
   15 March 2020.]

3.2

Social Distancing Is a Privilege
The Idea that This Virus Is an Equal-Opportunity Killer Must Itself Be Killed

Charles M. Blow

People like to say that the coronavirus is no respecter of race, class or country, that the disease COVID-19 is mindless and will infect anybody it can.[1]

In theory, that is true. But, in practice, in the real world, this virus behaves like others, screeching like a heat-seeking missile toward the most vulnerable in society. And this happens not because it prefers them, but because they are more exposed, more fragile and more ill.

What the vulnerable portion of society looks like varies from country to country, but in America, that vulnerability is highly intersected with race and poverty.

Early evidence from cities and states already shows that black people are disproportionately affected by the virus in devastating ways. As ProPublica reported, in Milwaukee County, Wis., as of Friday morning, 81 percent of the deaths were black people.[2] Black people make up only 26 percent of that county.

As for Chicago, WBEZ reported [on April 5, 2020] that "70 percent of COVID-19 deaths are black," and pointed out about surrounding Cook County, "While black residents make up only 23 percent of the population in the county, they account for 58 percent of the COVID-19 deaths."[3]

The Detroit News reported [on April 2, 2020], "At least 40 percent of those killed by the novel coronavirus in Michigan so far are black, a percentage that far exceeds the proportion of African-Americans in the Detroit region and state."[4]

If this pattern holds true across other states and cities, this virus could have a catastrophic impact on black people in this country.

And yet, we are still not seeing an abundance of news coverage or national governmental response that center on these racial disparities. Many states haven't even released race-specific data on cases and deaths. The federal government hasn't either.

Partly for this reason, we are left with deceptive and deadly misinformation. The perception that this is a jet-setters' disease, or a spring breakers' disease, or a "Chinese virus" as President Trump likes to say, must be laid to rest. The idea that this virus is an equal-opportunity killer must itself be killed.

And, we must dispense with the callous message that the best defense we have against the disease is something that each of us can control: We can all just stay home and keep social distance.[5]

As a report [in March 2020] by the Economic Policy Institute pointed out, "less than one in five black workers and roughly one in six Hispanic workers are able to work from home."[6]

As the report pointed out, "Only 9.2 percent of workers in the lowest quartile of the wage distribution can telework, compared with 61.5 percent of workers in the highest quartile."

If you touch people for a living, in elder care or child care, if you cut or fix their hair, if you clean their spaces or cook their food, if you drive their cars or build their houses, you can't do that from home.

Staying at home is a privilege. Social distancing is a privilege.

The people who can't must make terrible choices: Stay home and risk starvation or go to work and risk contagion.

And, this isn't just happening here, it is happening with poor people around the world, from New Delhi to Mexico City.

If they go to work, they must often use crowded mass transportation, because low-wage workers can't necessarily afford to own a car or call a cab.

Such is the life of the working poor, or those slightly above poverty, but still struggling. Our entire discussion around this virus is stained with economic elitism. In social media commentary about images of packed buses and crowds of delivery workers outside restaurants, people chastise black and brown people for not always being inside, but many of those doing the chastising do so from comfortable homes with sufficient money and food.

People can't empathize with what it truly means to be poor in this country, to live in a too-small space with too many people, to not have enough money to buy food for a long duration or anywhere to store it if they did. People don't know what it's like to live in a food desert where fresh fruit and vegetables are unavailable and nutrient-deficient junk food is cheap and exists in abundance.

People are quick to criticize these people for crowding into local fast food restaurants to grab something to eat. Not everyone can afford to order GrubHub or FreshDirect.

Furthermore, in a nation where too many black people have been made to feel that their lives are constantly under threat, the existence of yet another produces less of a panic. The ability to panic becomes a privilege existing among those who rarely have to do it.

I wholeheartedly encourage everyone who can to stay home, but I'm also aware enough to know that not everyone can or will, and that it is not simply a pathological disregard for the common good.

If you are sheltering in place in an ivory tower, or even a comfortable cul-de-sac or a smartly well-appointed apartment, and your greatest concern is boredom and leftover food, please stop scolding those scratching to survive.

Notes

1 Neil Vigdor, "Pastor Who Defied Social Distancing Dies after Contracting COVID-19, Church Says," *New York Times*, 14 April 2020.

2 Akilah Johnson and Talia Buford, "Early Data Shows African Americans Have Contracted and Died of Coronavirus at an Alarming Rate," *ProPublica*, 3 April 2020.

3 Elliott Ramos and María Inés Zamudio, "In Chicago, 70% of COVID-19 Deaths Are Black," *WBEZ*, 5 April 2020.

4 Craig Mauger and Christine MacDonald, "Michigan's COVID-19 Cases, Deaths Hit Blacks Disproportionately," *Detroit News*, 2 April 2020.

5 Vigdor, "Pastor Who Defied Social Distancing."

6 Elise Gould and Heidi Shierholz, "Not Everybody Can Work from Home," *Economic Policy Institute*, Working Economics Blog, 19 March 2020.

CASE STUDY

Going to a Park

Jack is 22 years old and recently graduated with a bachelor's degree in computer science. To save money while he pays back his student loans, he lives with his 79-year-old grandmother in a small house within a large and densely packed urban center.

In mid-February 2020, he began browsing Tinder. He met 23-year-old Karen, a server who lives nearby with three other roommates who work at the same restaurant, and they immediately hit it off. They began texting daily and talking on the phone nearly every night. Though both of them were initially hesitant to meet up in person with someone they'd met online, after a month of frequent conversations they came to trust each other and both desired to meet.

Unfortunately, the city issued stay-at-home orders on March 16, 2020, just a month after they'd first connected on Tinder. Since then, the city has directed residents to remain at home except for essential activities such as grocery shopping. Restaurants are allowed to remain open, but only for take-out and delivery. The city parks are open to walk through, but people are required to maintain at least six feet of separation from each other and are not allowed to sit or linger.

Jack knows that the city is discouraging people from getting together when they do not live in the same household, but he has been really looking forward to meeting Karen in person. He is desperate for human connection beyond the occasional hug from his grandmother. The stay-at-home orders have prevented him from seeing friends or colleagues, let alone going on dates, and Jack has felt the significant weight of depression as a result of these restrictions on social contact.

Jack is thinking of suggesting that he and Karen get take-out from Karen's favorite restaurant, Bar Agricole, and eat it in the park. He knows that people are not supposed to get within six feet of each other, but he has a blanket that would allow them to stay apart while enjoying their meal. Jack has heard on the news that the new disease, COVID-19, does not really affect people in their twenties, so he believes that meeting up with Karen would be relatively safe. He does not have any masks or gloves as the pandemic caught him by surprise. He had heard about it on the news months earlier, but he initially thought the outbreak was confined to East Asia. He was in disbelief when his city announced hundreds of cases and community spread.

Should Jack invite Karen to the picnic? Does he have any moral obligations to follow public health directives? Should considerations of mental health weigh into Jack's decision?

If Jack asks her to go on the picnic, should Karen accept? Are the moral obligations of Jack and Karen the same?

Do Jack and Karen have moral obligations to closely follow the news so as to ensure that they're aware of the disease's effects and of relevant public health directives? If Jack and Karen have learned as much as they can about the effects and spread of the disease, and they believe that the public health directives are more stringent than needed, does this in any way justify them in acting contrary to those directives?

QUESTIONS FOR REFLECTION

1. Are restrictive measures such as quarantines and physical distancing requirements morally justified in a pandemic? On what grounds? Is there a need to balance individual freedoms against concern for the public good, or does one of these always trump the other? Which moral values influence your answer?

2. Do individuals have moral obligations to adhere to restrictive measures? Why or why not? If a person fails to adhere to restrictions, is the government justified in punishing them?

3. If governments issue stay-at-home orders, do they thereby incur moral obligations to provide people with what is needed in order to comply? Which of the following is included in what is "needed"?

   a. Money for food and rent; safe housing for those who are homeless or precariously housed

   b. Guaranteed continuity of employment

   c. Heroin, alcohol, or other substances for drug-dependent people

   d. Internet access (especially in rural areas) so that people can continue working or learning from home

   e. Computers for children living in poverty so that they can continue learning from home

   f. Masks or other PPE

4
Scarce Resource Allocation

INTRODUCTION

In normal practice, doctors have a duty "to treat until there is evidence of harm or futility."[1] However, during the COVID-19 pandemic many hospitals have been overwhelmed beyond their surge capacity. Many patients experiencing sudden acute respiratory syndrome need breathing support from ventilators, but some hospitals don't have enough ventilators to go around. Health-care professionals are forced to shift from patient-centered care to population-centered care, in which they act as stewards for scarce resources. Doctors and other health-care providers are thus asked to make difficult decisions that will not only cost some patients their lives but also cause tremendous moral distress to those making the decisions.

Ethicists can help in these situations by providing clear moral guidance. When health-care professionals receive advice on how to ration scarce resources, they no longer have to bear the weight of these decisions alone. In this chapter, we examine some of the proposed criteria by which to ration scarce resources during a pandemic.

In the first of the included readings, a group of medical doctors and ethicists consider four moral values that could guide decisions around rationing: maximizing benefits, treating everyone equally, promoting and rewarding instrumental value, and giving priority to the worst off. The authors claim that maximizing benefits is the most important value during a pandemic and that this value can justify taking a patient off a ventilator in order to give it to someone else who will benefit more from the treatment. Angela Ballantyne notes that maximizing benefits will in some cases lead to unequal outcomes for different groups. An emphasis on benefits may disproportionally disadvantage those who are already marginalized in society, such as people with disabilities, people experiencing poverty, and elderly people. Ballantyne argues that these unjust outcomes give us reason not to emphasize the maximization of benefits when choosing criteria for resource allocation.

Jackie Leach Scully argues that assumptions about the overall health, quality of life, and social utility of people with disabilities may lead to discriminatory allocation decisions. Disabilities often do not impair health, and people with disabilities often assign higher ratings to their quality of life than do people without disabilities. Scully is particularly concerned with evaluations that require a health-care provider to rank a patient's usefulness to society, as this practice seems to undermine belief in the equal value of human life and may disadvantage people with disabilities. In the reading that follows, Joseph Fins responds to some of the disability criticisms that have targeted New York's guidelines for the allocation of ventilators. Fins argues that the criteria used by the New York task force were meant to be purely physiological and that the use of these physiological criteria divorces the decision-making process from any potential sources of bias.

Another criterion that some have proposed as a means of allocating scarce resources is age. Franklin G. Miller holds that age-based rationing is justified both because elderly persons have a very low chance of survival when removed from ventilators and because, even if they do survive, they have on average fewer remaining years to live than younger people. Shai Held argues to the contrary, claiming that the COVID-19 pandemic has exposed North America's disregard for and dehumanization of the elderly. Held proposes that our society is wrong to value people based on their assumed economic productivity and should instead understand the intrinsic moral value of each human life.

KEY TERMS

moral distress: the emotional residue that results from a situation in which a health-care professional knows the morally correct action to take but is prevented from doing so because of resource shortages or structural constraints.

overflow: in a disaster, when hospitals are overwhelmed, patients may be placed in overflow locations other than intensive care unit (ICU) beds. For example, patients might be placed in hallways, stadiums, or hotels.

surge capacity: the ability of a hospital (or health system) to go beyond the normal limits of its functioning, for example in a disaster, crisis, or epidemic.

triage: the process of deciding which patients get medical resources in a time of scarcity.

ventilator: a machine that is used to take over the oxygenation of blood when a person is no longer capable of breathing on their own.

NOTE

1   Kenny, Nuala (2020). "Emergency Triage of Health Resources and Moral Distress of Caregivers," *La Croix International*.

4.1

Fair Allocation of Scarce Medical Resources in the Time of COVID-19

Ezekiel J. Emanuel, Govind Persad, Ross Upshur, Beatriz Thome, Michael Parker, Aaron Glickman, Cathy Zhang, Connor Boyle, Maxwell Smith, and James P. Phillips

COVID-19 is officially a pandemic. It is a novel infection with serious clinical manifestations, including death, and it has reached at least 124 countries and territories. Although the ultimate course and impact of COVID-19 are uncertain, it is not merely possible but likely that the disease will produce enough severe illness to overwhelm health care infrastructure. Emerging viral pandemics "can place extraordinary and sustained demands on public health and health systems and on providers of essential community services."[1] Such demands will create the need to ration medical equipment and interventions.

Rationing is already here. In the United States, perhaps the earliest example was the near-immediate recognition that there were not enough high-filtration N95 masks for health care workers, prompting contingency guidance on how to re-use masks designed for single use.[2] Physicians in Italy have proposed directing crucial resources such as intensive care beds and ventilators to patients who can benefit most from treatment.[3,4] Daegu, South Korea—home to most of that country's COVID-19 cases—faced a hospital bed shortage, with some patients dying at home while awaiting admission.[5] In the United Kingdom, protective gear requirements for health workers have been downgraded, causing condemnation among providers.[6] The rapidly growing imbalance between supply and demand for medical resources in many countries presents an inherently normative question: How can too tight medical resources be allocated fairly during a COVID-19 pandemic?...

Ethical Values for Rationing Health Resources in a Pandemic

Previous proposals for allocation of resources in pandemics and other settings of absolute scarcity, including our own prior research and analysis, converge on four fundamental values: maximizing the benefits produced by scarce resources, treating people equally, promoting and rewarding instrumental value, and giving priority to the worst off.[7-12] Consensus exists that an individual person's wealth should not determine who lives or dies.[7-16] Although medical treatment in the United States outside pandemic contexts is often restricted to those able to pay, no proposal endorses ability-to-pay allocation in a pandemic.[7-16]

Each of these four values can be operationalized in various ways (Table 1). Maximization of benefits can be understood as saving the most individual lives or as saving the most life-years by giving priority to patients likely to survive longest after treatment.[7,9,11,12] Treating people equally could be attempted by random selection, such as a lottery, or by a first-come, first-served allocation.[7,11] Instrumental value could be promoted by giving priority to those who can save others, or rewarded by giving priority to those who have saved others in the past.[7,12] And priority to the worst off could be understood as giving priority either to the sickest or to younger people who will have lived the shortest lives if they die untreated.[7,11-13]

TABLE 1
Ethical Values to Guide Rationing of Absolutely Scarce Health Care Resources in a COVID-19 Pandemic

Ethical Values and Guiding Principles	Application to COVID-19 Pandemic
Maximize benefits	
Save the most lives	Receives the highest priority
Save the most life-years—maximize prognosis	Receives the highest priority
Treat people equally	
First-come, first-served	Should not be used
Random selection	Used for selecting among patients with similar prognosis

Promote and reward instrumental value (benefit to others)	
Retrospective—priority to those who have made relevant contributions	Gives priority to research participants and health care workers when other factors such as maximizing benefits are equal
Prospective—priority to those who are likely to make relevant contributions	Gives priority to health care workers
Give priority to the worst off	
Sickest first	Used when it aligns with maximizing benefits
Youngest first	Used when it aligns with maximizing benefits such as preventing spread of the virus

The proposals for allocation discussed above also recognize that all these ethical values and ways to operationalize them are compelling. No single value is sufficient alone to determine which patients should receive scarce resources.[7-16] Hence, fair allocation requires a multivalue ethical framework that can be adapted, depending on the resource and context in question.[7-16]

Who Gets Health Resources in a COVID-19 Pandemic?

These ethical values—maximizing benefits, treating equally, promoting and rewarding instrumental value, and giving priority to the worst off—yield six specific recommendations for allocating medical resources in the COVID-19 pandemic: maximize benefits; prioritize health workers; do not allocate on a first-come, first-served basis; be responsive to evidence; recognize research participation; and apply the same principles to all COVID-19 and non–COVID-19 patients.

Recommendation 1: In the context of a pandemic, the value of maximizing benefits is most important.[3,9,11,12,14-16] This value reflects the importance of responsible stewardship of resources: it is difficult to justify asking health care workers and the public to take risks and make sacrifices if the promise that their efforts will save and lengthen lives is illusory.[12] Priority for limited resources should aim both at saving the most lives and at maximizing improvements in individuals' post-treatment length of life. Saving more lives and more years of life is a consensus value across expert reports.[9,11,12] It is consistent both with utilitarian ethical perspectives that emphasize population outcomes and with non-utilitarian views that emphasize the paramount value of each human life.[17] There are many reasonable ways of balancing saving more lives against saving more years of life;[15] whatever balance between lives and life-years is chosen must be applied consistently.

Limited time and information in a COVID-19 pandemic make it justifiable to give priority to maximizing the number of patients that survive treatment with a reasonable life expectancy and to regard maximizing improvements in length of life as a subordinate aim. The latter becomes relevant only in comparing patients whose likelihood of survival is similar. Limited time and information during an emergency also counsel against incorporating patients' future quality of life, and quality-adjusted life-years, into benefit maximization. Doing so would require time-consuming collection of information and would present ethical and legal problems.[11,17] However, encouraging all patients, especially those facing the prospect of intensive care, to document in an advance care directive what future quality of life they would regard as acceptable and when they would refuse ventilators or other life-sustaining interventions can be appropriate.

Operationalizing the value of maximizing benefits means that people who are sick but could recover if treated are given priority over those who are unlikely to recover even if treated and those who are likely to recover without treatment. Because young, severely ill patients will often comprise many of those who are sick but could recover with treatment, this operationalization also has the effect of giving priority to those who are worst off in the sense of being at risk of dying young and not having a full life.[8,12,13]

Because maximizing benefits is paramount in a pandemic, we believe that removing a patient from a ventilator or an ICU bed to provide it to others in need is also justifiable and that patients should be made aware of this possibility at admission.[3,11,12,16,18] Undoubtedly, withdrawing ventilators or ICU support from patients who arrived earlier to save those with better prognosis will be extremely psychologically traumatic for clinicians—and some clinicians might refuse to do so. However, many guidelines agree that the decision to withdraw a scarce resource to save others is not an act of killing and does not require the patient's consent.[9,11,12,16,18] We agree with these guidelines that it is the ethical thing to do.[9] Initially allocating beds and ventilators according to the value of maximizing benefits could help reduce the need for withdrawal.

Recommendation 2: Critical COVID-19 interventions—testing, PPE, ICU beds, ventilators, therapeutics, and vaccines—should go first to front-line health care workers and others who care for ill patients and who keep critical infrastructure operating, particularly workers who face a high risk of infection and whose training makes them difficult to replace.[10] These workers should be given priority not because they are somehow more worthy, but because of their instrumental value: they are essential to pandemic response.[10,11] If physicians and nurses are incapacitated, all patients—not just those with COVID-19—will suffer greater mortality and years of life lost. Whether health workers who need ventilators will be able to return to work is uncertain, but giving them priority for ventilators recognizes their assumption of the high-risk work of saving others, and it may also discourage absenteeism.[11,19] Priority for critical workers must not be abused by prioritizing wealthy or famous persons or the politically powerful above first responders and medical staff—as has already happened for testing.[20] Such abuses will undermine trust in the allocation framework.

Recommendation 3: For patients with similar prognoses, equality should be invoked and operationalized through random allocation, such as a lottery, rather than a first-come, first-served allocation process. First-come, first-served is used for such resources as transplantable kidneys, where scarcity is long-standing and patients can survive without the scarce resource. Conversely, treatments for coronavirus address urgent need, meaning that a first-come, first-served approach would unfairly benefit patients living nearer to health facilities. And first-come, first-served medication or vaccine distribution would encourage crowding and even violence during a period when social distancing is paramount. Finally, first-come, first-served approaches mean that people who happen to get sick later on, perhaps because of their strict adherence to recommended public health measures, are excluded from treatment, worsening outcomes without improving fairness.[16] In the face of time pressure and limited information, random selection is also preferable to trying to make finer-grained prognostic judgments within a group of roughly similar patients.

Recommendation 4: Prioritization guidelines should differ by intervention and should respond to changing scientific evidence. For instance, younger patients should not be prioritized for COVID-19 vaccines, which prevent disease rather than cure it, or for experimental post- or pre-exposure prophylaxis. COVID-19 outcomes have been significantly worse in older persons and those with chronic conditions.[21] Invoking the value of maximizing saving lives justifies giving older persons priority for vaccines immediately after health care workers and first responders. If the vaccine supply is insufficient for patients in the highest risk categories—those over 60 years of age or with coexisting conditions— then equality supports using random selection, such as a lottery, for vaccine allocation.[7,11] Invoking instrumental value justifies prioritizing younger patients for vaccines only if epidemiologic modeling shows that this would be the best way to reduce viral spread and the risk to others.

Epidemiologic modeling is even more relevant in setting priorities for coronavirus testing. Federal guidance currently gives priority to health care workers and older patients,[22] but reserving some tests for public health surveillance (as some states are doing) could improve knowledge about COVID-19 transmission and help researchers target other treatments to maximize benefits.[23]

Conversely, ICU beds and ventilators are curative rather than preventive. Patients who need them face life-threatening conditions. Maximizing benefits requires consideration of prognosis—how long the patient is likely to live if treated—which may mean giving priority to younger patients and those with fewer coexisting conditions. This is consistent with the Italian guidelines that potentially assign a higher priority for intensive care access to younger patients with severe illness than to elderly patients.[3,4] Determining the benefit-maximizing allocation of antivirals and other experimental treatments, which are likely to be most effective in patients who are seriously but not critically ill, will depend on scientific evidence. These treatments may produce the most benefit if preferentially allocated to patients who would fare badly on ventilation.

Recommendation 5: People who participate in research to prove the safety and effectiveness of vaccines and therapeutics should receive some priority for COVID-19 interventions. Their assumption of risk during their participation in research helps future patients, and they should be rewarded for that contribution. These rewards will also encourage other patients to participate in clinical trials. Research participation, however, should serve only as a tiebreaker among patients with similar prognoses.

Recommendation 6: There should be no difference in allocating scarce resources between patients with COVID-19 and those with other medical conditions. If the COVID-19 pandemic leads to absolute scarcity, that scarcity will affect all patients, including those with heart failure, cancer, and other serious and life-threatening conditions requiring prompt medical attention. Fair allocation of resources that prioritizes the value of maximizing benefits applies across all patients who need resources. For example, a doctor with an allergy who goes into anaphylactic shock and needs life-saving intubation and ventilator support should receive priority over COVID-19 patients who are not front-line health care workers....

Conclusions

Governments and policy makers must do all they can to prevent the scarcity of medical resources. However, if resources do become scarce, we believe the six recommendations we delineate should be used to develop guidelines that can be applied fairly and consistently across cases. Such guidelines can ensure that individual doctors are never tasked with deciding unaided which patients receive life-saving care and which do not. Instead, we believe guidelines should be provided at a higher level of authority, both to alleviate physician burden and to ensure equal treatment. The described recommendations could shape the development of these guidelines.

References

1 Pandemic influenza plan: 2017 update. Washington, DC: Department of Health and Human Services, 2017 (https://www.cdc.gov/flu/pandemic-resources/pdf/pan-flu-report-2017v2.pdf).
2 Strategies for optimizing the supply of N95 respirators. Atlanta: Centers for Disease Control and Prevention, 2020 (https://www.cdc.gov/coronavirus/2019-ncov/hcp/respirators-strategy/index.html).

3 Vergano M, Bertolini G, Giannini A, et al. Clinical Ethics Recommendations for the Allocation of Intensive Care Treatments, in Exceptional, Resource-Limited Circumstances. Italian
Society of Anesthesia, Analgesia, Resuscitation, and Intensive Care (SIAARTI). March 16,
2020 (http://www.siaarti.it/SiteAssets/News/COVID19%20-%20documenti%20SIAARTI/
SIAARTI%20-%20Covid-19%20-%20Clinical%20Ethics%20Reccomendations.pdf).

4 Mounk Y. The extraordinary decisions facing Italian doctors. Atlantic. March 11, 2020
(https://www.theatlantic.com/ideas/archive/2020/03/who-gets-hospital-bed/607807/).

5 Kuhn A. How a South Korean city is changing tactics to tamp down its COVID-19 surge.
NPR. March 10, 2020 (https://www.npr.org/sections/goatsandsoda/2020/03/10/812865169/
how-a-south-korean-city-is-changing-tactics-to-tamp-down-its-covid-19-surge).

6 Campbell D, Busby M. 'Not fit for purpose': UK medics condemn COVID-19 protection.
The Guardian. March 16, 2020 (https://www.theguardian.com/society/2020/mar/16/
not-fit-for-purpose-uk-medics-condemn-covid-19-protection).

7 Persad G, Wertheimer A, Emanuel EJ. Principles for allocation of scarce medical interventions. Lancet 2009;373:423–31.

8 Emanuel EJ, Wertheimer A. Public health: who should get influenza vaccine when not all
can? Science 2006;312:854–55.

9 Biddison LD, Berkowitz KA, Courtney B, et al. Ethical considerations: care of the critically ill and injured during pandemics and disasters: CHEST consensus statement. Chest
2014;146:4 Suppl:e145S-e155S.

10 Interim updated planning guidance on allocating and targeting pandemic influenza vaccine during an influenza pandemic. Atlanta: Centers for Disease Control and Prevention,
2018 (https://www.cdc.gov/f lu/pandemic-resources/national-strategy/ planning-guidance/
index.html).

11 Rosenbaum SJ, Bayer R, Bernheim RG, et al. Ethical considerations for decision making
regarding allocation of mechanical ventilators during a severe influenza pandemic or other
public health emergency. Atlanta: Centers for Disease Control and Prevention, 2011 (https://
www.cdc.gov/od/science/integrity/phethics/docs/Vent_Document_Final_Version.pdf).

12 Zucker H, Adler K, Berens D, et al. Ventilator allocation guidelines. Albany: New York State
Department of Health Task Force on Life and the Law, November 2015 (https://www.health.
ny.gov/regulations/task_force/reports_publications/docs/ventilator_guidelines.pdf).

13 Christian MD, Sprung CL, King MA, et al. Triage: care of the critically ill and injured during
pandemics and disasters: CHEST consensus statement. Chest 2014;146:4 Suppl:e61S-e74S.

14 Responding to pandemic influenza—the ethical framework for policy and planning.
London: UK Department of Health, 2007 (https://webarchive.nationalarchives.gov.
uk/20130105020420/http://www.dh.gov.uk/prod_consum_dh/groups/dh_digitalassets/@
dh/@en/documents/digitalasset/dh_080729.pdf).

15 Toner E, Waldhorn R. What US hospitals should do now to prepare for a COVID-19 pandemic. Baltimore: Johns Hopkins University Center for Health Security, 2020 (http://www.
centerforhealthsecurit y.org/cbn/2020/cbnreport-02272020.html).

16 Influenza pandemic—providing critical care. North Sydney, Australia: Ministry of Health,
NSW, 2010 (https://www1.health.nsw.gov.au/pds/ActivePDSDocuments/PD2010_028.pdf).

17 Kerstein SJ. Dignity, disability, and lifespan. J Appl Philos 2017;34:635–50.

18 Hick JL, Hanfling D, Wynia MK, Pavia AT. Duty to plan: health care, crisis standards of care,
and novel coronavirus SARS-CoV-2. NAM Perspectives. March 5, 2020 (https://nam.edu/
duty-to-plan-health-care-crisis-standards-of-care-and-novel-coronavirus-sars-cov-2/).

19 Irvin CB, Cindrich L, Patterson W, Southall A. Survey of hospital healthcare personnel
response during a potential avian influenza pandemic: will they come to work? Prehosp
Disaster Med 2008;23:328–35.

20 Biesecker M, Smith MR, Reynolds T. Celebrities get virus tests, raising concerns of inequality. Associated Press March 19, 2020 (https://apnews.com/b8dcd1b369001d5a70eccdb1f 75ea4bd).

21 Wu Z, McGoogan JM. Characteristics of and important lessons from the coronavirus disease 2019 (COVID-19) outbreak in China: summary of a report of 72 314 cases from the Chinese Center for Disease Control and Prevention. JAMA 2020 February 24 (Epub ahead of print).

22 Updated guidance on evaluating and testing persons for coronavirus disease 2019 (COVID-19). Atlanta: Centers for Disease Control and Prevention, March 8, 2020 (https://emergency.cdc.gov/han/2020/han00429.asp).

23 COVID-19 sentinel surveillance. Honolulu: State of Hawaii Department of Health, 2020 (https://health.hawaii.gov/docd/covid-19-sentinel-surveillance/).

4.2

ICU Triage
How Many Lives or Whose Lives?

Angela Ballantyne

Bioethicists around the world have been asked to advise on the goals and methods of triage protocols. Estimates suggest 5% of COVID-19 cases will require ICU care.[1] The key ethical tension is between utility and equity. There are other relevant principles of fair allocation such as reciprocity for frontline workers who have taken extraordinary risks; and a "fair innings" to prioritize those who are younger on the grounds that they have lived a shorter proportion of their natural life span. I leave these aside for now, because the major tension is between utility and equity.

The World Health Organization defines health equity as preventing remediable differences among groups of people, whether those groups are defined socially, economically, or demographically.[2] We cannot simultaneously prioritize utility (saving the most lives) and equity (avoiding unjust discrimination).

These values are direct trade-offs.[3] We can save more lives or we save a more diverse group of lives. There is no perfect algorithm but we need to identify an acceptable balance.

Several influential bioethicists have argued that is it simply obvious that the "many" matters more than the "who":

- "in a situation where resources are overwhelmed, and choices cannot be avoided, the ethical balance must shift to emphasising benefit...this will mean prioritising intensive care for those patients who have the highest chance of surviving."[4]
- "Priority for limited resources should aim both at saving the most lives and at maximizing improvements in individuals' post-treatment length of life. Saving more lives and more years of life is a consensus value across expert reports."[5]
- "As a basic rule, we try to act in such a way that the largest number of people survive, because that is in the public interest."[6]

According to these positions, the value of saving lives is a substantially more weighty ethical consideration than the value of equal outcomes. It is unsurprising that guidelines based on utility have already elicited legal challenge on the grounds of disability discrimination.[7] Implicit cognitive biases will likely lead clinical decision-makers to unconsciously and unfairly discriminate against older persons or persons with disability.[8] Some of the proposed triage tools add explicit barriers. Jackie Leach Scully argues that current triage guidelines are an "...indicator of our ongoing inability as a society to consider people with disabilities as equal members of the community, with equal human and civil rights, equal claims to citizenship, and equal moral agency."[9]

In this blog I consider the impact of a utility-focused triage approach on social and ethnic health disparities and question why equity has been so quickly de-prioritized. ICU triage tools cannot be expected to fix the problems of long-standing health disparities. But that doesn't mean we should uncritically accept the mantra of utility.

There will be a point at which the prospect of a patient's survival in ICU will be so low that admittance would amount to a failure to responsibly steward public resources. But there is significant ground between maximizing ICU survival and senselessly throwing away resources. This middle ground should include at least some space for deprioritising utility in favor of giving a wider range of people a shot at ICU. Contrary to the dominant position described above, I argue that equity and justice are critical public interests that must be protected.

Of course those justifying prioritization of utility don't endorse discrimination. But in reality, an ethical approach aimed at maximizing lives saved results in prioritizing certain social groups. The easy lives to save will be those of people who already enjoy social privilege. As a population, younger, white, wealthy people will be more likely to derive benefit from the ICU resources and survive because they enjoy, on average, higher baseline health status.

Comorbidities are not evenly distributed amongst the population. Underlying health status correlates with privilege based ethnicity and wealth.[10] Current evidence suggests that people with hypertension, cardiovascular disease, chronic obstructive pulmonary disease (COPD), and cancer are more likely to die from severe COVID-19.[11] In New Zealand for example prevalence of multimorbidity (two or more conditions) is higher for Māori (13.4%) and Pacific ethnic groups (13.8%) than for NZ Europeans (7.6% prevalence).[12] Multimorbidity is also more common for people in areas of higher socioeconomic deprivation. Māori aged 45 and over have a COPD hospitalisation rate over 3.5 times that of non-Māori.[13] When you plug the clinical status of individuals into an ICU triage tool aimed at maximising population survival rates you will get results that reflect these social and ethnic divisions.

Exposure to coronavirus may also vary by socio-economic status. The ability to socially isolate is a luxury. According to US cell phone data, high income demographic groups have reduced their geographic scope of movement more significantly than lower income groups.

Prior epidemics in New Zealand have had disproportionate impact on Māori and Pacific peoples.[14] This wasn't as a result of differential access to ICU, but probably does reflect vulnerabilities relating to underlying health status and access to medical care. The first ICUs were established in the late 1950s so access to ICU was not a relevant factor in the 1918 pandemic; and ICU access was not triaged during the 2009 pandemic in New Zealand. During the 1918 influenza pandemic, Māori in New Zealand died at eight times the rate of Europeans.[15] During the 2009 H1N1 pandemic the mortality rate was 2.6 times higher for Māori and 5.8 times higher for Pacific peoples than European New Zealanders.[16]

Maximising the number of lives saved is a function of (1) prognosis (chance of survival) and (2) length of time to benefit (how long each patient is likely to need ICU care).[17] A key problem for utilitarianism has always been the accuracy of predictions. Standard scoring systems for ICU mortality are designed to predict capacity to benefit from ICU care. These include APACHE-II, sequential organ failure assessment (SOFA), and Simplified Acute Physiology Score. SOFA for example assesses the severity of the patient's clinical state based on function/dysfunction of six major organ systems.[18] But how reliable are these scoring systems in predicting survival of severe COVID-19 patients in ICU?

In China, the overall case-fatality rate (CFR) was 2.3%; but the CFR was higher for patients with pre-existing comorbid conditions—10.5% for cardiovascular disease, 7.3% for diabetes, 6.3% for chronic respiratory disease, 6.0% for hypertension, and 5.6% for cancer.[19] The CFR was 49% among critical cases, but detailed information about critically ill COVID-19 patients is scarce.[20]

Analysis of emerging UK data published [on 27 March 2020] found that 7 COVID-19 patients with severe comorbidities survived ICU (41.2%) whereas 10 died (58.8%).[21] Is this data sufficient, either in quality or differential outcome, to suggest that those with even severe comorbidities should be denied access to

ICU? If we are going to deny specific patients access to ICU on the grounds of population utility we need a high degree of confidence in the clinical evidence.

Given this uncertainty, what can we do? I am not a health provider and not in a position to interpret the emerging clinical evidence or speak to the reliability of different ICU scoring systems. But as bioethicists are invited to consult on these triage tools we need to be asking hard questions about the reliability of the screening measures used to exclude certain patients.

Where there is uncertainty, we should err on the side of broader rather than stricter clinical criteria; meaning a wider range of patients get a shot at ICU, even where this is likely to be less efficient overall. Screening measures that include Quality Adjusted Life Years (QALYs) must be avoided as these are inherently biased against persons with disabilities.[22] When resources are limited we need to allow time constrained ICU trials, and generate protocols for withdrawing ICU care.[23] These are important mechanisms to give more people access to ICU. The following approach goes some way towards limiting the impact of comorbidities on access criteria:

> To address concerns about compounding injustices associated with systematic disadvantage and the arbitrariness of comorbidities, and unlike other approaches that have been proposed for ICU triage in a disaster, the scoring system described here affects patients whose comorbidities are so serious that they are expected to live no more than 12 months even with successful ICU treatment.[24]

Regardless of the specific number of patients who survive severe COVID-19, we will need to tell a story about the values that guided us as a community in a time of crisis. The narratives that emerge during this pandemic will have a lasting legacy in bioethics. Public interest requires the responsible use of resources. But this does not exclusively entail maximizing utility. There is public interest in reaffirming human rights, the value of diversity, promoting fairness, and resisting entrenched privilege.

Notes

1 Wei-jie Guan et al., "Clinical Characteristics of Coronavirus Disease 2019 in China," *New England Journal of Medicine*, 30 April 2020.
2 World Health Organization, "Equity," www.who.int/healthsystems/topics/equity/en/.
3 John Broome, "Fairness, Goodness and Levelling Down," in *Summary Measures of Population Health*, ed. J.L. Murray et al. (Geneva: World Health Organization, 2002).
4 Dominic J.C. Wilkinson, "ICU Triage in an Impending Crisis: Uncertainty, Pre-emption and Preparation," *Journal of Medical Ethics*, 1 April 2020.
5 Ezekiel J. Emanuel et al. "Fair Allocation of Scarce Medical Resources in the Time of COVID-19," *New England Journal of Medicine*, 23 March 2020.

6 Dr. Georg Marckmann, quoted in Andrea Grunau, "Coronavirus and Ethics: 'Act so that most people survive,'" DW.com, 24 March 2020.

7 Disability Rights Education & Defense Fund, "Preventing Discrimination in the Treatment of COVID-19 Patients," 25 March 2020.

8 Elizabeth N. Chapman et al., "Physicians and Implicit Bias: How Doctors May Unwittingly Perpetuate Health Care Disparities," *Journal of General Internal Medicine* 28, no. 11 (November 2013); Joseph Stramondo, "COVID-19 Triage and Disability: What NOT to Do," www.bioethics.net, 30 March 2020.

9 Jackie Leach Scully, "Disablism in a Time of Pandemic: Some Things Don't Change," *International Journal of Feminist Approaches to Bioethics Blog*, 1 April 2020.

10 Donna Cormack et al., "Investigating the Relationship between Socially-Assigned Ethnicity, Racial Discrimination and Health Advantage in New Zealand," *PLoS One* 8, no. 12 (31 December 2013); R.B. Harris et al., "The Relationship between Socially-Assigned Ethnicity, Health and Experience of Racial Discrimination for Māori: Analysis of the 2006/07 New Zealand Health Survey," *BMC Public Health* 13 (13 September 2013).

11 Zunyou Wu and Jennifer M. McGoogan, "Characteristics of and Important Lessons from the Coronavirus Disease 2019 (COVID-19) Outbreak in China," *JAMA* 323, no. 13 (24 February 2020).

12 James Stanley et al., "Epidemiology of Multimorbidity in New Zealand: A Cross-Sectional Study Using National-Level Hospital and Pharmaceutical Data," *BMJ Open* 8 (2018): e021689, doi:10.1136/bmjopen-2018-021689.

13 "Tatau Kahukura: Māori Health Statistics," New Zealand Ministry of Health, 2 August 2018.

14 Emma Espiner, "New Zealand Must Learn Lessons of 1918 Pandemic and Protect Māori from COVID-19," *The Guardian*, 25 March 2020.

15 K. Drennan et al., "Impact of Pandemic (H1N1) 2009 on Australasian Critical Care Units," *Critical Care and Resuscitation* 12, no. 4 (December 2010).

16 Nick Wilson et al., "Relatively High Mortality for Māori and Pacific Peoples in the 2009 Influenza Pandemic and Comparisons with Previous Pandemics," https://www.otago.ac.nz/wellington/otago024539.pdf.

17 Wendy Rogers and Stacy Carter, "Ethical Considerations Regarding Allocation of Ventilators/ICU Beds during Pandemic-Associated Scarcity."

18 Yehudit Aperstein et al., "Improved ICU Mortality Prediction Based on SOFA Scores and Gastrointestinal Parameters," *PLoS One* 14, no. 9 (30 September 2019).

19 Wu and McGoogan, "Characteristics."

20 Xiaobo Yang et al., "Clinical Course and Outcomes of Critically Ill Patients with SARS-CoV-2 Pneumonia in Wuhan, China: A Single-Centered, Retrospective, Observational Study," *The Lancet Respiratory Medicine* 8, no. 5 (24 February 2020).

21 "Report on 775 Patients Critically Ill with COVI-19," *Intensive Care National Audit & Research Centre*, 27 March 2020.

22 Rogers and Carter, "Ethical Considerations."

23 D.J. Wilkinson and J. Savulescu, "Knowing When to Stop: Futility in the ICU," *Current Opinion in Anesthesiology* 24, no. 2 (April 2011).

24 E. Lee Daugherty Biddison, et al., "Too Many Patients…: A Framework to Guide Statewide Allocation of Scarce Mechanical Ventilation During Disasters," *CHEST Journal* 155, no. 4 (April 2019).

4.3

Disablism in a Time of Pandemic

Jackie Leach Scully

The COVID-19 pandemic is currently accompanied by a parallel outbreak of bioethical and clinical ethical discussion offering guidance for the difficult decisions that healthcare professionals and others face as the pandemic develops. Right at the moment there is a strong focus on the *ethics of triage*. In countries affected by COVID-19, healthcare professionals are having or will have to decide which patients get access to life-saving critical care—in the case of COVID-19 that means intensive care beds and ventilators—when there is not enough for everyone in need. They want guidance on how to make those decisions in the most morally justifiable way. Just as much, patients, families and the general public want to know the basis on which such decisions are being made.

In all the published guidance that has appeared [in the early weeks of the pandemic], one thing is disturbingly clear. Many of these resources have shown a worrying degree of prejudice against disabled people, or disablism. Protocols from Alabama and Tennessee have been namechecked here.[1] While it is easy to see in these evidence of a straightforward disvaluing of the lives of people with disabilities—and at worst, the seizure of a golden opportunity to get rid of burdensome people—in reality something more complex is going on. It's equally unacceptable, but understanding offers better ways of challenging it.

Disablist Assumptions
Three overlapping but conceptually distinct disablist assumptions critically endanger people with disabilities in a situation of clinical care triage:

- first, there are assumptions about the overall health status of disabled people;
- second, assumptions about disabled people's quality of life; and
- finally, assumptions about disabled people's social utility, which in fact only becomes relevant if there is confusion about the role it plays (or shouldn't play) in critical care decision-making.

As background, it's important to recognise that most triage protocols use probable clinical outcome as the primary decision-making criterion. In essence this comes down to the likelihood that the treatment will save the life of a person who would otherwise not recover. Being able to recover without it, or being pretty certain to die despite it, are both reasons for not receiving treatment. When there are many people who are equally in need of and likely to benefit from a treatment in short supply, we attempt to refine the clinical criteria, i.e., to make them more stringent, always in order to identify the core of people most likely to benefit from treatment, in the fairest possible way. ("Fairest possible" begs a lot of questions, and several different principles have been suggested in the bioethical literature: I won't go into them here.)

A key factor is a person's *background health status*, because some underlying conditions are already known to significantly decrease the chance of recovery from the severe form of COVID-19—including hypertension, cardiovascular disease, chronic obstructive pulmonary disease, and cancer.[2] But disability by itself, however, often has no impact on health. People with visual and hearing impairments for example, or intellectual disability, can be just as healthy and therefore as likely to recover with treatment as anyone else. In other words, disability shouldn't automatically be used as a proxy for compromised health.

What makes the ethical terrain here more complicated is that some disabling conditions *do* involve health issues that are relevant to chance of recovery—if lung function is affected, for example, or if long-term medication has led to seriously raised blood pressure. But even here, it is important to recognize that individual differences mean global rules (of the "no one with cystic fibrosis to be placed on ventilation" kind) could easily be unjust. This is important because both bioethics and medical ethics have dismayingly bad track records of oversimplifying the diversity hidden in "disability" to the point of uselessness.

The second set of assumptions concern predicted longer-term *quality of life*. Although there is general consensus that critical care decisions should primarily be based on predicted outcome, in many cases the wording of guidelines leaves it unclear whether considerations about quality of life are implicitly or explicitly being drawn in as well. And using predicted quality of life to make allocation decisions in a broadly disablist society generates a profound bias against people with disabilities. We know from abundant empirical evidence that people without disabilities tend to take it as a given that disability inescapably leads to life being worse, while disabled people on the whole rate their own quality of life as at least as good as anyone else's. One reason for this discrepancy is the simple difficulty of projecting oneself imaginatively into a very unfamiliar kind of life, without experiencing *different* as *lesser*. Triage guidance that, even implicitly, draws on assumptions about the quality of the saved life is in danger of codifying an unarticulated belief that "they can't actually enjoy life like that."

The third issue is even more complex, because it involves both prejudice and a slippage of triage criteria. Major ethical tensions arise when decision makers start to reach beyond the likelihood of benefit to the individual and towards some idea of "*social utility*," in other words how valuable that person, if saved, will be to society. Triaging by social utility is the shift that should probably concern us the most: it's also the one most likely to be resisted by patients and families, and to cause moral distress in healthcare professionals.

Even this is complicated, because many people nevertheless agree that in disaster or health emergency it makes moral as well as practical sense to prioritise the care of frontline medical staff, because it benefits everyone to have them healthy and working again as rapidly as possible. In situations of massive social collapse, there will be arguments for prioritizing people who can offer other vital services as well. (Of course, this would not necessarily discriminate against disability: a disabled person with experience in engineering or food production would be more socially useful than, say, a professor of bioethics.) But the SARS-CoV-2 pandemic is *not* social collapse; and there is no ethical justification for making critical care decisions on the basis of factors like profession, or personal circumstances, or assumptions about the productivity or value to society of a disabled person.

Discriminatory Norms

The assumptions I've discussed above (about disabled people's health, quality of life, and social utility) are formed by a framework of ideas about norms. Disability activism and scholarship have helped to identify and challenge the powerful biomedical, cultural, political and economic forces that delineate what modern western societies consider to be normal for human form, function and behavior. Nevertheless, it's clear that often the reasoning of the published guidance on triage has been shaped by unacknowledged norms and unexamined assumptions about life lived with disability and the "value" (for want of a better word) of disabled people.

For example, the UK National Institute for Health and Care Excellence's COVID-19 Rapid Guidance[,] ...released on 21 March 2020, recommended prioritizing critical care resources based on something called the Clinical Frailty Scale.[3] The Guidance said that the CFS was used because it helped "to identify patients who are at increased risk of poor outcomes and who may not benefit from critical care interventions." However, as patient groups and representatives quickly pointed out, the CFS's categorization of different levels of frailty used criteria that don't necessarily play any role in clinical outcome for COVID-19 or, indeed, in overall quality of life, and could mistakenly be applied to people with stable disabilities otherwise in perfectly good health. For instance, the Guidelines suggest using CFS level 5 or more as one factor in making critical care decisions: yet the description of "frailty" at CFS level 5 would apply to many healthy people with disabilities, including people with learning disabilities, autism, cerebral palsy and so on.

In response to criticism, four days after the original NICE guidelines were released they were modified to note that "The CFS should not be used in younger people, people with stable long-term disabilities (for example, cerebral palsy), learning disabilities or autism" and that assessments should be individualised and holistic. This swift response is admirable. Nevertheless, these and other guidelines show a worrying lack of awareness that norms aren't universal: that a lot of people who don't fit the social norm of independent ability to dress, move around, or make autonomous decisions—whose dependence is more obvious than other people's—are nevertheless healthy and lead flourishing lives that are no worse or better than anyone else's.

Despite the last half century of progress in recognizing disabled people's rights, and irrespective of what public and policy might say openly, these problematic responses are an indicator of our ongoing inability as a society to consider people with disabilities as equal members of the community, with equal human and civil rights, equal claims to citizenship, and equal moral agency. This fundamental inability has potentially catastrophic consequences for disabled people in the COVID-19 global health emergency.

Some Recommendations

- In all cases, critical care guidance should include not just the *criteria* for triage decisions, but explanation of the *reasoning behind them.*
- Disability status should not be used as a simple proxy for health status.
- Critical care decisions should be based on knowledge of an individual's personal medical history, not on assumptions about background health status or quality of life (and preferably not relying solely on medical records, which are notoriously error-prone).
- Critical care decisions should be scrupulous in excluding considerations of broad social utility.
- And critical care guidance should acknowledge openly that disabled people are to be treated as equally valuable and worthy of care as others.

Notes

1 Ari Ne'eman, "I Will Not Apologize for My Needs," *The New York Times*, 23 March 2020.
2 Zunyou Wu and Jennifer M. McGoogan, "Characteristics of and Important Lessons from the Coronavirus Disease 2019 (COVID-19) Outbreak in China," *JAMA*, 24 February 2020.
3 National Institute for Health and Care Excellence, "COVID-19 Rapid Guideline: Critical Care in Adults NICE Guideline [NG159]," 20 March 2020.

4.4

Disabusing the Disability Critique of the New York State Task Force Report on Ventilator Allocation

Joseph J. Fins

I am a member of the New York State Task Force on Life and the Law and helped write its 2015 guidelines on the allocation of ventilators during a public health emergency. The position outlined by the Task Force report has been a point of confusion in the media, and it was notably misrepresented by Ari Ne'eman, a disability activist, in an op-ed in *The New York Times*.[1] The confusion is understandable given the legacy of discrimination against people with disabilities.

While I cannot speak for the New York State Task Force on Life and the Law, as an academic, I can share with colleagues the approach that I believe we outlined. As I understand our work, we sought to achieve a physiologically based methodology centering on the Sequential Organ Failure Assessment (SOFA) score to prioritize ventilator allocation once a public health emergency was upon us. Seeking refuge in the objectivity of the SOFA score, we sought to achieve a fair allocation of resources divorced from other socially-constructed determinants that could introduce bias and disadvantage those on the margins of society.

Once a declaration has been made of a crisis standards of care, as defined by the 2012 Institute of Medicine report,[2] patients would be triaged into four color-coded categories based on their SOFA scores: Blue, Green, Red, and Yellow. Simply stated, those designated as Blue would not likely survive the acute infection despite maximal efforts. Green were those who were sick and did not need a ventilator. Red patients were most likely to survive if they received a ventilator. Yellow was an intermediate class between Red and Blue.

We didn't recommend allocation decisions based on advanced age, as we believed that patients' *physiologic* age was baked into SOFA scores, which track the functionality of several organ systems. The Task Force also intended to avoid discriminating against individuals with disabilities. When such discrimination takes place, a disability that has no bearing on outcome is used to deny care. This bias—often reflective of unrelated notions of social worth—can be subtle: a medical condition associated with a disability is used as rationale for rationing even though it would not affect outcome. An example of *crypto-discrimination* might be the heart conditions associated with Down syndrome even when these conditions had no bearing on survival. Discrimination based on disability is alleged to have occurred in Washington State. In response, the US Department of Health and Human Services' Office for Civil Rights in Action has issued a bulletin citing federal law that prohibits discrimination against people with disabilities.[3]

Discrimination against people with disabilities creeps easily into medical decision-making. I made this point in *Rights Come to Mind: Brain Injury, Ethics and the Struggle for Consciousness*[4] and in an op-ed in the same *New York Times* disability series that hosted the essay by Ne'eman.[5] In these forums, I used a disability rights prism to advocate for individuals with disorders of consciousness. I do not believe, however, that the recommendations in the Task Force report discriminate against people with disabilities. The report seeks to disentangle disability from one's ability to survive respiratory failure necessitating mechanical ventilation. I vividly recall a heated discussion during the Task Force deliberations in which we debated what would constitute the pool of ventilators that would be subject to allocation. Would someone who used a ventilator due to a chronic disability lose that ventilator to the collective?

The late Adrienne Asch, a disability scholar and bioethicist who was a member of the Task Force, helped us distinguish a ventilator in chronic use to maintain the health of someone with a pre-existing lung condition from a ventilator which was used in response to an acute pandemic. With her typical eloquence and vigor, Asch argued that the chronic ventilator was part and parcel of that person. As such it was not subject to being commandeered in a crisis. It was theirs, not the collective's. However, if that same person was admitted to the hospital and needed to make a claim on a more sophisticated ventilator because of a new severe illness, then they would be subject to the same assessment as everyone else. That was discriminating but *not* discriminatory. Sadly, Asch passed away in 2013, two years before the Task Force report was published.

The report isn't a perfect methodology. It will be amended by circumstances and necessity. But I am glad we were able to do much hard work before the current crisis struck. New Yorkers and others who may draw upon it are fortunate that the report was not an ad hoc effort drawn up in the heat of the moment.

Notes

1 Ari Ne'eman, "I Will Not Apologize for My Needs," *The New York Times*, 23 March 2020.

2 Institute of Medicine, *Crisis Standards of Care: A Systems Framework for Catastrophic Disaster Response* (The National Academies Press, 2012).

3 HHS Office for Civil Rights in Action, "BULLETIN: Civil Rights, HIPAA, and the Coronavirus Disease 2019 (COVID-19)," 28 March 2020.

4 Joseph J. Fins, *Rights Come to Mind* (Cambridge University Press, 2015).

5 Joseph J. Fins, "Brain Injury and the Civil Right We Don't Think About," *The New York Times*, 24 August 2017.

4.5

Why I Support Age-Related Rationing of Ventilators for COVID-19 Patients

Franklin G. Miller

The COVID-19 pandemic raging around the world is raising health-related ethical issues from the micro level of individuals and families to the macro level of governments and societies. The pressing issue of availability of mechanical ventilators spans the territory. Reflecting on that issue demonstrates that bioethics is *personal* and *political*. As a 71-year-old bioethicist, I recently drew up an advance directive specifically for the possibility that I might have to go to the hospital with COVID-19, and I am writing this essay to explain why I consider rationing mechanical ventilation based on age to be one morally relevant criterion.

As the surge of patients presses on hospitals, the resources of intensive care beds and mechanical ventilators are likely to be insufficient to treat all who may need them to have a chance at survival. Who should get access to these scarce resources when all can't be served? Who will die to make way for others who might have a chance to live?

Within the context of medical ethics, with its focus on the clinician-patient dyad, no ethical issue is more fraught than the allocation of scarce medical technology. Indeed, it was on the radar of philosophers and theologians at the very beginning of bioethics as a field of study, more than 50 years ago, in particular in the context of the novel intervention of dialysis for end-stage renal disease.

In normal times, outside of a health crisis, intensive care beds and technology are properly allocated first-come-first-served. This is unsatisfactory when the existing supply is outstripped by demand, as is occurring, or likely to soon occur, in the COVID-19 pandemic. In such a context, rationing of some sort becomes morally imperative. What criteria should govern access to ventilators?

A short essay does not afford space for a systematic argument in favor of age as one, but not the only, criterion for rationing the use of ventilators in the context of the COVID-19 pandemic, especially for doing justice to various objections that would be raised. Nevertheless, the key ethical considerations can be outlined. Some patients suffering from COVID-19 develop a progressive pneumonia, which may rapidly lead to severe respiratory insufficiency; for these patients, mechanical ventilation, often for two weeks or more, may become necessary to give them a chance of survival.

While outcomes data are meager at this point, they suggest a grim prospect for elderly patients needing mechanical ventilation. A single medical center in Wuhan, China described intensive care outcomes for 52 patients.[1] Of that total, 37 patients received mechanical ventilation, and 30 of them, 80%, died during the 28-day follow-up. Of 10 patients aged 70 and older, only one survived. A much larger data set reporting outcomes for 1,591 patients in ICUs in Lombardy, Italy between February 20 and March 18, 2020, demonstrated considerably higher rates of mortality depending on age: 29% for those 61–70; 40% for those 71–80; and 55% for those 81 and older.[2] However, many patients in those age groups remained in the ICU at the time the study was completed. For the 22 patients aged 81 and over, 12 had died (55%); 2 had been discharged (9%); and 8 (36%) remained in the ICU. If half of those remaining in the ICU in that age group subsequently died, the overall mortality rate would be 73%; if all of them died, it would be 91%.

In addition to older patients having a relatively poor prognosis, the number of years of life that they have had the opportunity to experience supports an age criterion for rationing ventilators. Other things being equal, the young have much more to lose from death than the elderly. I would suggest that an initial age criterion for rationing ventilators when the demand outstrips the supply is a cut-off of 80. Eighty years of age is just above the average life expectancy in the US, which is 79 years old.[3] It seems fair to say that people who have reached that milestone have enjoyed an opportunity to live a complete life. On average, not many years of life with relatively good health and functioning are left to those aged 80.

If demand for ventilators keeps growing and further outstrips supply, I believe it could be justifiable as a matter of policy to forgo mechanical ventilation for all patients 70 years of age and older who have a medical condition that puts them at elevated risk of death, such as chronic renal disease, cardiovascular disease, diabetes, and chronic lung disease. Finally, in a yet more dire shortage I believe the age limit could be set at 70, regardless of a patient's overall medical condition. This stringent rationing policy would include me. I view myself as having lived a complete life. Losing a relatively small chance of survival and recovery to a tolerable quality of life seems to me a reasonable sacrifice in favor of younger patients, and consistent with promoting the common good in the extraordinary societal situation posed by the current pandemic.

To be sure, the surge of COVID-19 patients in need of mechanical ventilation in the US might not overwhelm available resources, such that implementing an age criterion for rationing becomes justifiable; however, the situation in other countries might be relevantly different.

Some people will object to my proposal on the grounds that I am endorsing age discrimination. But what matters is whether using age as a rationing criterion is reasonable and fair.

A policy of rationing that adopts age as a criterion can be morally tolerable only if elderly patients who must forgo mechanical ventilation receive adequate palliative care. In the pressure to save lives during a pandemic, palliative care might become neglected; however, failure to provide it abandons patients to unnecessary suffering and bad deaths. The right of all patients to receive medically-indicated, life-sustaining treatment, and the duty of clinicians to provide it, may need to be limited during a pandemic. In contrast, palliative care is a moral imperative for all critically ill patients.

Notes

1 X. Yang, Y. Yu, J. Xu, et al., "Clinical Course and Outcomes of Critically Ill Patients with SARS-CoV-2 Pneumonia in Wuhan, China: A Single-Centered, Retrospective, Observational Study" [published online ahead of print, 24 February 2020] [published correction appears in *The Lancet Respiratory Medicine* 8, no. 4 (April 2020): e26], *The Lancet Respiratory Medicine*, 2020.

2 Giacomo Grasselli et al., "Baseline Characteristics and Outcomes of 1591 Patients Infected with SARS-CoV-2 Admitted to ICUs of the Lombardy Region, Italy," *Journal of the American Medical Association* 323, no. 16 (6 April 2020).

3 Elizabeth Arias and Jiaquan Xu, "United States Life Tables, 2017," *National Vital Statistics Reports* 68, no. 7 (24 June 2019).

4.6

The Staggering, Heartless Cruelty toward the Elderly
A Global Pandemic Doesn't Give Us Cause to Treat the Aged Callously

Shai Held

Crises can elicit compassion, but they can also evoke callousness. Since the outbreak of the coronavirus pandemic, we've witnessed communities coming together (even as they have sometimes been physically forced apart), and we've seen individuals engaging in simple acts of kindness to remind the sick and quarantined that they are not forgotten. Yet from some quarters, we've also seen a degree of cruelty that is truly staggering.

Earlier today, a friend posted on Facebook about an experience he'd just had on the Upper West Side of Manhattan: "I heard a guy who looked to be in his 20s say that it's not a big deal cause the elderly are gonna die anyway. Then he and his friend laughed…Maybe I'm lucky that I had awesome grandparents and maybe this guy didn't but what is wrong with people???" Some have tried to dress up their heartlessness as generational retribution. As someone tweeted at me earlier today, "To be perfectly honest, and this is awful, but to the young, watching as the elderly over and over and over choose their own interests ahead of climate policy kind of feels like they're wishing us to a death they won't have to experience. It's a sad bit of fair play."

Notice how the all-too-familiar rhetoric of dehumanization works: "The elderly" are bunched together as a faceless mass, all of them considered culprits and thus effectively deserving of the suffering the pandemic will inflict upon them. Lost entirely is the fact that the elderly are individual human beings, each with a distinctive face and voice, each with hopes and dreams, memories and regrets, friendships and marriages, loves lost and loves sustained. But *they* deserve to die—and as for us, we can just go about our business.

It is bad enough if we remain indifferent to the plight of our elders; it is far worse to dress up our failings as moral indignation.

As a rabbi and theologian watching this ethical train wreck, I find myself thinking about the biblical mandate to "honor your father and mother." The Hebrew word usually translated as "honor," *kabed*, comes from a root meaning "weight." At the deepest level, then, the biblical command is thus to treat the elderly as weighty. Conversely, the Bible prohibits "cursing" one's parents. The Hebrew word usually translated as "curse," *tekalel*, derives from a root meaning "light." At bottom, then, the biblical proscription is on treating the elderly lightly, as if they are inconsequential.

Why do I say "the elderly"? In its biblical context, the obligation to honor parents is a command given to grown children (as are the Ten Commandments more broadly—you don't tell children not to commit adultery nor to covet their neighbors' fields). When you are an adult, the Bible instructs, you must not abandon the elderly. Giving voice to a pervasive human fear, the Psalmist prays, "Do not cast me off in old age; when my strength fails, do not forsake me!"

What does it say about our society that people think of the elderly so dismissively—and moreover, that they feel no shame about expressing such thoughts publicly? I find myself wondering whether this colossal moral failure is exacerbated by the most troubled parts of our cultural and economic life. When people are measured and valued by their economic productivity, it is easy to treat people whose most economically productive days have passed as, well, worthless.

From a religious perspective, if there is one thing we ought to teach our children, it is that our worth as human beings does not depend on or derive from

SCARCE RESOURCE ALLOCATION

what we do or accomplish or produce; we are, each of us, infinitely valuable just because we are created in the image of God. We mattered before we were old enough to be economically productive, and we will go on mattering even after we cease to be economically productive.

Varied ethical and religious traditions find their own ways to affirm an elemental truth of human life: The elderly deserve our respect and, when necessary, our protection. The mark of a decent society is that it resists the temptation to spurn the defenseless. It is almost a truism that the moral fabric of a society is best measured by how it treats the vulnerable in its midst—and yet it is a lesson we never seem to tire of forgetting. "You shall rise before the aged and show deference to the old," the Bible says—look out for them and, in the process, become more human yourself.

CASE STUDY

Ventilator Shortages: Who Should Live?

Forty-four-year-old Janet Greene is a single mother of two young children who went on government assistance early in the pandemic after losing her job as a restaurant server. Janet lives in a rural area with limited medical resources. One day, she began to experience headaches, shortness of breath (dyspnea), and a loss of smell (anosmia). Within a week, she was gasping for air and having difficulty remaining conscious. She was admitted to the ICU in her local community hospital, where she tested positive for COVID-19.

Dr. Achebe was concerned by Janet's oxygen levels and so administered an epinephrine injection and an albuterol inhalation. Dr. Achebe gave Janet oxygen through a nasal tube, but her levels continued to fall and Janet risked hypoxemia. He thought she might soon need to be intubated and placed on a ventilator. The hospital has two ventilators; however, both of them are occupied by other patients who've tested positive for COVID-19 and are being treated by other physicians. Dr. Achebe knows that his hospital's pandemic triage policy allows for the removal of patients from ventilators when their condition is not likely to improve.

Dr. Bashar is treating Xiao-ping, a retired 70-year-old Asian-American man with six grandchildren. Xiao-ping was in excellent health before he came down with COVID-19, and Dr. Bashar believes Xiao-ping's prognosis is good if he remains on the ventilator but that he has a high probability of dying if it were removed.

Dr. Connor is treating Yasmine, a 22-year-old single woman who is also in a serious medical state. Yasmine has type-1 diabetes, liver disease, and autoimmune disorder. These conditions don't normally have a negative effect on Yasmine's quality of life, but they put her at increased risk of mortality from COVID-19. Dr. Connor is reluctant to remove Yasmine from the ventilator because she will most likely have many happy years ahead of her if she survives.

Dr. Achebe knows that another person in the community is also using a ventilator due to a severe but permanent respiratory condition unrelated to the coronavirus. Zola is a man with disabilities who has the ventilator attached to his wheelchair. He does not currently have COVID-19, but due to his other health conditions he can survive for only an hour without the ventilator. Dr. Achebe thinks Janet will need the ventilator for several days.

What should Dr. Achebe do? Which moral principles or allocation criteria would favor the removal of the ventilator from one of the other patients in order to help Janet? If Dr. Achebe believes that the ventilator should be removed from one of the other patients and he presents this argument to his colleagues, how should Dr. Bashar and Dr. Connor respond? Are Dr. Bashar's and Dr. Connor's obligations toward their own patients outweighed by other obligations (to public health, to adherence to rationing protocols, etc.)? If the doctors determine that they should remove the ventilator from one of the other patients in order to help Janet, what should they tell the family of the patient from whom the ventilator is removed?

QUESTIONS FOR REFLECTION

1. What moral values ought to govern decisions around resource allocation? What priority would you give to each? Why? Are there any groups of people that would be disadvantaged by the values and priority you've chosen?

2. Ballantyne and Scully criticize some of the proposed standards for resource allocation on the grounds that they may disadvantage certain groups, such as disabled people, ethnic minorities, and people of lower socio-economic status. Do you find their arguments convincing? Why or why not? Could the criteria proposed by Emanuel et al. be adjusted in response to Ballantyne's and Scully's arguments?

3. Are there other groups that may potentially be disadvantaged by an emphasis on maximizing benefits when rationing scarce medical resources?

4. Is Fins's response to the disability criticism successful?

5. Is it morally justified to use age as a criterion (or even the sole criterion) when making decisions about scarce resource allocation? Adjudicate between Miller and Held.

5
Justice

INTRODUCTION

There are many different forms of justice (see the key terms below), but this chapter focuses mainly on what I will call "social" justice. Social justice can operate at a domestic or a global level. Within a society, social justice obtains when there is equity among different social groups (defined by race, class, gender, sexual orientation, (dis)ability status, age, ethnicity, etc.). Those who defend a social justice approach seek to eliminate the oppression, exploitation, disadvantage, powerlessness, and barriers placed upon these groups. At the global level, advocates of social justice seek to remove inequities among nations. Those who work toward achieving social justice are concerned with distributions of social goods, but they also attend to more intangible concerns that are not parcelled out and distributed, such as respect.[1]

Past pandemics have served to exacerbate existing social inequities, and there is evidence that the same is occurring with COVID-19. Shaun Ossei-Owusu argues that social inequities in the United States that existed before the current pandemic created classes of people who are now more vulnerable to the disease. Government policies and citizen indifference have led to systemic inequalities, and these inequalities mean that the poor, the racialized, and those with disabilities are more likely to come into contact with SARS-CoV-2 than are people of privilege. And members of those disadvantaged groups face greater risk of mortality if they develop COVID-19, as they often live without the same levels of health care and insurance.

This chapter concludes with a reading by Alex Broadbent and Benjamin T.H. Smart, who note that policies that work in Europe and North America may be less effective or inappropriate in an African context. Yet, as they point out, the World Health Organization (WHO) has not issued region-specific advice for addressing COVID-19 in Africa. African leaders are therefore pressured to conform to WHO measures that have been designed elsewhere, even when the costs of those measures might outweigh their benefits.

KEY TERMS

equality: occurs when individuals or groups are treated in the same way. Equal treatment will not always lead to equity because some groups might need different treatment in order to have a fair chance.

equality of opportunity: when all individuals or groups have the same initial chance to succeed. Some proponents of equality of opportunity argue that a resulting inequality of outcome may be just so long as it is the result of a difference in individual effort or performance rather than a difference in opportunity.

equality of outcome: when the distribution of a good is equal to all persons and is not dependent on individual effort or merit.

equity: occurs when individuals or groups all receive fair treatment. Inequities are not mere inequalities; they are *unjust* inequalities.

health inequities: unjust inequalities of health status, whether at the domestic or the international level.

justice: a basic moral concept that takes many forms.

> **distributive justice:** when goods are allotted using an appropriate principle such as need, merit, ability to pay, or social utility. In the context of COVID-19, distributive justice may have bearing on the allocation of scarce resources.

> **restorative justice:** when amends are made for harms done to others. Financially compensating the victim of a crime is an example of an attempt at restorative justice.

> **retributive justice:** involves praise and blame, reward and punishment. "Eye-for-an-eye" punishment is a form of retributive justice.

> **social justice:** equity among different social groups (as defined by race, class, gender, sexual orientation, (dis)ability status, age, ethnicity, etc.).

social determinants of health: the social and economic factors that influence a person or group's health in positive or negative ways. For example, people living in poverty or in polluted areas will often experience health problems as a result. The social determinants of health include income and income distribution, social status, education and literacy, unemployment and job security, physical environments, employment and working conditions, childhood experiences, food insecurity, housing, social exclusion, social safety networks, access to health services, sexism, racism, ableism, and access to land.

NOTE

1 Iris Marion Young (1990), *Justice and the Politics of Difference* (Princeton University Press).

5.1

Coronavirus and the Politics of Disposability

Shaun Ossei-Owusu

In the final chapter, "The Space Traders," of his 1992 book *Faces at the Bottom of the Well: The Persistence of Racism*, Derrick Bell, Harvard Law School's first tenured black professor, described a fictive world eerily similar to the one we know today. Local and federal governments ostensibly had no money. "Decades of conservative, laissez-faire capitalism had emptied the coffers of all but a few of the very rich," the narrator says. Because of a host of poor choices, the country "was struggling to survive like any third-world nation," and financial exigencies "curtailed all but the most necessary services." The parallels are acute: "the environment was in shambles, as reflected by the fact that the sick and elderly had to wear special masks whenever they ventured out-of-doors."

In the story, English-speaking extraterrestrial beings land on the shores of New Jersey and offer to solve everything: gold to bail out companies, chemicals to unpollute the environment. The country could have this deal for one sweet price: "all the African Americans who lived in the United States." This was the central, controversial claim in Bell's science fiction: that white people would sell black people to aliens for the right price. The story concludes with a successful trade. Twenty million black men, women, and children are stripped to just one undergarment, lined up, chained, and whisked away, like many of their ancestors' centuries before.

Bell's story lays bare the politics of disposability. But unlike the cosmos of the Space Traders, the world of coronavirus is not simply black/white. It is white and non-white;[1] poor and not poor;[2] essential and non-essential; white collar and blue collar;[3] Asian and not Asian;[4] undocumented and citizen;[5] able-bodied and sick;[6] young and elderly;[7] first-generation higher ed students and their wealthier counterparts;[8] the free and imprisoned;[9] celebrities with access to instant testing and plebeians;[10] red states and blue states;[11] and countless other binaries. From these overlapping inequities we get a glimpse of who is disposable: the people who occupy the wrong category. The scholar and cultural critic Henry Giroux analyzes this politics in his book *Against the Terror of Neoliberalism* (2008). "It is a politics in which the unproductive (the poor, weak and racially marginalized) are considered useless and therefore expendable," he writes—and "in which entire populations are considered disposable, unnecessary burdens on state coffers, and consigned to fend for themselves."

Tragically, demographic data about COVID-19 deaths are beginning to bear this vision out. On [6 April 2020,] Kaiser Health News reported that "A Disproportionate Number Of African-Americans Are Dying, But The US Has Been Silent On Race Data."[12] Seventy percent of those who have died from coronavirus in Chicago are black.[13] [The week of 29 March to 3 April] saw calls from a range of politicians,[14] journalists,[15] and scholars[16] for more fine-grained data than has been made available thus far. But for many observers, who was being impacted was the *first* question on their mind. Beyond the latest numbers, we have other data points: history, what is visible from news and experience, and media accounts. These are imperfect, but they supply some information, and the implications are grim.

The people whose disposability is on widest display are those who work in immediate-risk industries: the financially precarious service workers, the health care workers tasked with "equity work."

This is certainly *not* to say—as some multiracial groups of conspiracy theorists allege—that there is some sinister grandmaster plot afoot to harm vulnerable populations.[17] In Bell's allegory intent can often be a sideshow, if not an outright distraction. The truth is more banal: systemic social inequalities have made some groups more vulnerable than others, and the question of intent is irrelevant. As a criminal law professor, I teach my students that intent matters, but in some instances it does not. In this context, malfeasance,[18] misguided policies,[19] and indifference[20] suffice. Moreover, while government is the easy and most identifiable culprit, popular complicity is at play here too, which makes this version of disposability different from Bell's telling.[21]

The people whose disposability is on widest display are those who work in immediate-risk industries. The financially precarious service workers out with the epidemiological wolves so the rest of society can buy groceries.[22] The health care workers plastered on the news, who labor in a profession that tasks minority and women nurses, physician assistants, and technicians with what sociologist Adia Harvey Wingfield calls "equity work": labor that makes health institutions more available to marginalized groups.[23] The homeless population, which was already noticeable in US cities, is now more conspicuous because of their inability to shelter in place.[24]

Then there are the undocumented agricultural workers in the west and south-west who can't work on Zoom like their white-collar counterparts and have now become more precious in a country that has insisted on calling them illegal.[25] There are Native Americans—some of whom have been facing a long-standing water crisis[26]—who have uniquely high rates of diseases that make COVID-19 more lethal.[27] There are the Asian Americans who have been subject to hate crimes since this virus surfaced in the US.[28] And there are the residents in poorly serviced public housing projects in places like Chicago,[29] Baltimore,[30] and my native South Bronx, where 2,000 public housing residents woke up to no water during an epidemic that requires vigilant hand washing.[31]

The recent history of other US disasters is also telling. The Chicago Heatwave of 1995 killed more than 700 people, mostly poor and elderly, and necessitated refrigerated trucks for dead corpses[32] in ways that are similar to New York now.[33] A decade later, Hurricane Katrina took the lives of more than 1,800 people in Louisiana, many of whom were poor and could not leave their homes as advised. Poor people in New York City face the same today: they do not have the benefit of escaping to second homes in Long Island and New England.[34] And then there was Hurricane Maria, which was a little more than eighteen months ago. That disaster, which killed approximately 3,000 people in Puerto Rico, elicited similar criticisms of the federal government's slow response and accusations that the death count was severely understated.[35] Jason Cortés has described President Trump's paper-towel-throwing spectacle during his visit to Puerto Rico as "the American commander-in-chief [choosing] to toss disposable paper to disposable people."[36]

On Palm Sunday [5 April], Surgeon General Jerome Adams gave an ominous warning. "This is going to be the hardest and the saddest week of most Americans' lives, quite frankly," he cautioned. "This is going to be our Pearl Harbor moment, our 9/11 moment. Only, it's not going to be localized, it's going to be happening all over the country. And I want America to understand that."[37] But who exactly will be dispensed with? It certainly won't be all of us. Collective pronouns—the "we" and "our" and "us" of public discourse—are dangerously comforting. They give the impression of equal susceptibility, while celebrities and other prominent figures gain access to testing and top-flight health care.[38] COVID-19 is not discriminatory as a biological matter, but history and available accounts indicate that the epidemiological fallout will be weighty and uneven.

During the debates about the *Affordable Care Act*, hysteria emerged around government-run "death panels": committees of doctors who would ration care and decide who would receive treatment. This alarm ignored the long history of rationing and unequal access to health care—the subject of Beatrix Hoffman's book *Rights and Rationing in the United States Since 1930* (2012)—but it echoes legitimate dismay about bureaucrats making decisions about who lives and who dies. People with disabilities, racial minorities, undocumented immigrants, prisoners, and the poor did not figure prominently into the frenzy around death panels, but they have reason to be worried now. The uninsured, elderly, and an ever-growing portion of the middle class should be added to that list.

Social science data has already shown that African Americans are often denigrated, disregarded, and disbelieved by medical professionals when they claim they are in pain.[39] Where will they fit in the treatment queues? Can we rest assured that American doctors will not take a cue from those in Italy, who deprioritized the lives of coronavirus patients who are chronically ill, disabled, or elderly?[40] What about the Latinx folk who constitute a third of uninsured people in the country?[41] Bioethical scenarios usually reserved for grad school seminars are likely to be actualized.

Rural whites have been relatively safe from the virus for now (but not its economic impact[42]). Most live in the approximately 1,300 counties that have no confirmed cases and where social distancing is ordinary.[43] But many of these counties are also medical deserts unequipped to handle this virus. If COVID-19 creeps into these locales, as it has in Albany, Georgia,[44] will this group of people—many of whom perceive themselves to be "strangers in their own land," as the title of the sociologist Arlie Hochshild's 2018 book put it—be disregarded, too? And if the virus does not make its way to rural America, what does that say about the disposability of everyone else?

Bell's "Space Traders" struck a nerve because it highlighted the vulnerability of an entire class of people. The difference now is that the people being sacrificed extend beyond African Americans, and responsibility can be tethered not only to government but to the private sector, the media, and the parts of the general public. The outcome of this story is uncertain. But when the dust settles, as in all US disasters, there will be a tale to tell of who mattered and who was sacrificed.

Notes

1 Deborah Barfield Berry, "Health Issues for blacks, Latinos and Native Americans May Cause Coronavirus to Ravage Communities," *USA Today*, 30 March 2020.

2 Derek Thompson, "The Coronavirus Will Be a Catastrophe for the Poor," *Atlantic*, 20 March 2020.

3 Abigail Hess, "Coronavirus Highlights the Inequality of Who Can—and Can't—Work from Home," *CNBC*, 4 March 2020.

4 Lauren Aratani, "'Coughing while Asian': Living in Fear as Racism Feeds Off Coronavirus Panic," *Guardian*, 24 March 2020.

5 Lulu Garcia-Navarro, "What Happens If Undocumented Immigrants Get Infected with Coronavirus?," *NPR*, 29 March 2020.

6 Daniel Morain and Anita Chabria, "Coronavirus Frays the Safety Net for People with Severe Disabilities, Leaving Many at Risk," *Los Angeles Times*, 5 April 2020.

7 "People Who Are at Higher Risk for Severe Illness," Centers for Disease Control and Prevention, 14 May 2020.

8 Karin Fischer, "When Coronavirus Closes Colleges, Some Students Lose Hot Meals, Health Care, and a Place to Sleep," *Chronicle of Higher Education*, 11 March 2020.

9 Anna Flagg and Joseph Neff, "Why Jails Are So Important in the Fight Against Coronavirus," *The Marshall Project*, 31 March 2020.

10 Chris Cwik, "NBA Explains Why Its Players Have Access to Coronavirus Tests while General Public Does Not," *Yahoo! Sports*, 18 March 2020.

11 Ronald Brownstein, "Red and Blue America Aren't Experiencing the Same Pandemic," *Atlantic*, 20 March 2020.

12 "A Disproportionate Number of African-Americans Are Dying, but the US Has Been Silent on Race Data," *Kaiser Health News*, KHN Morning Briefing, 6 April 2020.

13 Samantha Michaels, "70 Percent of People Killed in Chicago by the Coronavirus Are Black," *Mother Jones*, 5 April 2020.

14 Aaron Morrison, "Elizabeth Warren and Ayanna Pressley Are Calling for Racial Data on Coronavirus Tests," *Boston.com*, 30 March 2020.

15 Charles M. Blow, "The Racial Time Bomb in the COVID-19 Crisis," *New York Times*, 1 April 2020.

16 Ibram X. Kendi, "Why Don't We Know Who the Coronavirus Victims Are?," *Atlantic*, 1 April 2020.

17 Nick Bilton, "Coronavirus Is Creating a Fake-News Nightmarescape," *Vanity Fair*, 2 March 2020.

18 Kevin Johnson and Ledyard King, "Justice Department Launches Inquiry of Senators Who Sold Large Chunks of Stock before Coronavirus Market Slide," *USA Today*, 30 March 2020.

19 Ross Barkan, "Cuomo Helped Get New York into This Mess," *Nation*, 30 March 2020.

20 Caitlin Oprysko, "Fauci Warns against Coronavirus Indifference among Young People," *Politico*, 15 March 2020.

21 Melissa Wiley, "Photos of Packed Beaches, Bikeways, and Hiking Trails Show How People Are Ignoring Coronavirus Social-Distancing Mandates around the World," *Business Insider*, 24 March 2020.

22 Alan Berube and Nicole Bateman, "Who Are the Workers Already Impacted by the COVID-19 Recession?," *Brookings*, 3 April 2020.

23 Adia Harvey Wingfield, *Flatlining: Race, Work, and Health Care in the New Economy* (University of California Press, 2019).

24 Samantha Melamed, "'It's Heartbreaking': Coronavirus Puts Philly Homeless Services in Survival Mode," *Philadelphia Inquirer*, 19 March 2020.

25 Andrea Castillo, "Farmworkers Face Coronavirus Risk: 'You Can't Pick Strawberries over Zoom'," *Los Angeles Times*, 1 April 2020.

26 Bill Chappell, "Coronavirus Cases Spike in Navajo Nation, Where Water Service Is Often Scarce," *NPR*, 26 March 2020.

27 Dana Hedgpeth, Darryl Fears, and Gregory Scruggs, "Indian Country, where Residents Suffer Disproportionately from Disease, Is Bracing for Coronavirus," *Washington Post*, 4 April 2020.

28 Alexandra Kelley, "Attacks on Asian Americans Skyrocket to 100 per Day during Coronavirus Pandemic," *The Hill*, 31 March 2020.

29 Mick Dumke, "The Chicago Housing Authority Was Slow to Protect Residents during the Coronavirus Outbreak," *ProPublica Illinois*, 30 March 2020.

30 Annie Rose Ramos, "Coronavirus in Maryland: Low-Income Communities Hit Especially Hard by COVID-19," *CBS Baltimore*, 1 April 2020.

31 Michael Gartland and Larry McShane, "Rattled Tenants in Bronx Housing Project Wake Up with No Running Water, Raising Fears of Coronavirus Infection among Its 2,000 Residents," *New York Daily News*, 4 April 2020.

32 Eric Klinenberg, quoted in "Dying Alone: An interview with Eric Klinenberg," *University of Chicago Press* website, https://press.uchicago.edu/Misc/Chicago/443213in.html

33 Justine Coleman, "FEMA Sending Refrigerator Trucks to NYC for Coronavirus Deaths," *The Hill*, 30 March 2020.

34 Alexandra Sternlicht, "As Wealthy Depart for Second Homes, Class Tensions Come to Surface in Coronavirus Crisis," *Forbes*, 29 March 2020.

35 Keith Naughton, "Coronavirus: It's Time to Get Real about the Misleading Data," *The Hill*, 1 April 2020.

36 Jason Cortés, "Puerto Rico: Hurricane Maria and the Promise of Disposability," *Capitalism Nature Socialism*, vol. 29, no. 3, 2018.

37 William Cummings, "'This Is Going to Be Our Pearl Harbor': Surgeon General Warns USA Faces Worst Week of Coronavirus Outbreak," *USA Today*, 5 April 2020.

38 Robin Young and Allison Hagan, "While Some Wait for COVID-19 Tests, the Wealthy Cut the Line," *WBUR*, 19 March 2020.

39 Janice A. Sabin, "How We Fail Black Patients in Pain," *AAMC*, 6 January 2020.

40 Ariana Eunjung Cha, "Spiking US Coronavirus Cases Could Force Rationing Decisions Similar to Those Made in Italy, China," *Washington Post*, 15 March 2020.

41 Edward Berchick, "Most Uninsured Were Working-Age Adults," *United States Census Bureau*, 12 September 2018.

42 Jacob Bonge, Kirk Maltais, and Jesse Newman, "Coronavirus Hits Already Frail US Farm Economy," *Wall Street Journal*, 21 March 2020.

43 Morgan Lee and Nicky Forster, "Counties without Coronavirus Are Mostly Rural, Poor," *Associated Press*, 29 March 2020.

44 Graham Rapier, "How a Small Georgia City Far from New York Became One of the Worst Coronavirus Hotspots in the Country," *Business Insider*, 7 April 2020.

5.2

Why a One-Size-Fits-All Approach to COVID-19 Could Have Lethal Consequences

Alex Broadbent and Benjamin T.H. Smart

Suppose you had the choice between two health policies, A and B. Policy A would result in the death of a lot of elderly people. Policy B would result in the death of a lot of children, especially infants. Which would you choose?

Right now we are facing a choice between more or less drastic measures to slow the spread of COVID-19, a virus which, [as of March 23, 2020], has yet to claim a life under 10, and claims very few lives under 30, with the risk rising exponentially with age.[1] We are putting in place measures that will lead to malnutrition and starvation for millions of people, and for these horrors, children and especially infants are the most at risk. And very many of those infants are born, and will die, in Africa.[2]

Yet there is little discussion of the consequences for human health of the measures we are taking.[3] Nor is there discussion of how the major differences between Africa and America, Europe and Asia might matter. The World Health Organization (WHO) website contains no technical guidance on how African governments should approach their considerably different contexts. The advice is the same globally, but the context is not.

Failure to recognise that one size does not fit all could have lethal consequences in this region, maybe even more lethal than those of the virus itself.

Social Distancing May Cost Lives in Africa

In Africa, millions will starve if the global economy enters a protracted downturn. We must ask whether the number will be more than COVID-19 will kill in a region where only 6.09% of the population is over 65.[4]

After the 2008 recession, 1 billion people were malnourished, and 5 million more children were hungry in 2010 than they would have been if the recession had not happened.[5] We are only seeing the start of the economic disaster, and therefore the health disaster, that is going to engulf us as a consequence of social distancing measures.

And it's not just the plunge of some abstract stock market. Tourism employs 1 in 23 employed South Africans.[6] It has evaporated overnight. Bars and restaurants are empty, and, where they serve alcohol, must close early or limit numbers. Football has been shut for the season, and football clubs will go bust. And so on.

Unemployment in South Africa was already nearly 30% in the fourth quarter of 2019.[7] The government lacks both the means and the competence to swiftly dish out grants to SMEs, such as the GBP10,000.00 (about South African R200,000.00) offered by the British government.[8] South African SMEs are already vulnerable. Their employees mostly have no savings, no access to credit (creating hospitable waters for loan sharks[9]), limited assets, and a support network consisting of people in the same boat. Mass unemployment means mass poverty, which means mass starvation.

The crunch question is this: what is the case fatality rate of social distancing in Africa? We have no idea; but that is the figure that should be considered when implementing social distancing measures. The scientific community, including both epidemiologists and economists working together, should be putting as much effort into estimating that case fatality rate as into estimating it for COVID-19.

Social Distancing Might Not Work in Africa

It's not even clear that the social distancing measures will curb the spread of disease here. We know from award winning work on HIV transmission by South African epidemiologists that local social context can neuter a health intervention that is effective elsewhere.[10] So it may be with social distancing.

In a South African township, living conditions are extremely crowded. Socialising is unavoidable. You might as well tell people to emigrate to Mars. In the bubonic plague, the aristocracy left London for the countryside; the poor of London could not isolate themselves, and so they died.[11] This may be our situation.

It is similarly fantastical to expect people who cannot afford food—as will soon be the case for many more—to practice personal hygiene. You can't eat soap. If you are starving, you won't buy it.

Thus the major components of the recommended public health measures—social distancing and hygiene—are extremely difficult to implement effectively in much of Africa. The net effect of measures that seek to enforce social distancing may thus be to prevent people from working, without actually achieving the distancing that would slow the spread of the virus. If that is true, then we must consider whether we would be better off without them.

Not all these measures are the same, and nor are preventive measures an all-or-nothing measure. Some degree of social distancing may be possible. Elbow greetings may slow things down. But it's a fantasy to suppose that the virus can be contained anywhere, and the cost of measures must be proportioned to their likely benefit. The cost of an elbow greeting is low, but the cost of shutting a school is huge.

But even if social distancing here will "flatten the curve," will it make a difference?[12] The logic of flattening the curve is to bring the peak of the pandemic (the highest number of sick at any one time) down to a manageable level. But this assumes access to healthcare in the first place.

In much of Africa, public healthcare is inaccessible to a huge proportion of the population. Without a miraculously fast overhaul of the continent's healthcare provision, flattening the curve will make no difference to the majority. Cute as the meme is, its logic does not apply to much of Africa.

What about the Children?

Children evoke strong emotions in most of us. Those with children may be worried about their welfare. But children are at very low direct risk from the virus,[13] although of course they are at indirect risk from the economic consequences of pandemic and the death of elderly care-givers.[14] And, in a famine, they are at very high risk of malnutrition and starvation.

We, personally, have elderly relatives whom we care about deeply. But would we actively move children who are otherwise at a minimal risk into a high risk situation, in an attempt to prolong the life of some of those elderly? Would we do so when the effectiveness of those measures is questionable, and the economic effects of those measures (famine) also puts the elderly themselves at risk?

We don't know. It depends on the data. But we do believe that this is a conversation that we must be brave enough to have.

Many leaders are doubtless aware of their dilemma, but their ability to express this and their ability to make choices is restricted, as the treatment of British leadership shows. In Africa, it's questionable whether leaders have a political choice, given intense pressure from an international community that isn't thinking about the differences of the African context, and a WHO offering no region-specific technical advice.

Leaders need to be given the space to say shocking things, to be upfront about what might go wrong, to change their minds in the face of new evidence, and to pick the lesser of two evils.[15]

Doctors face such choices every day, and they are horrible. But they are unavoidable. Without a proper estimation of the costs as well as the benefits of the measures currently being implemented, no rational assessment of their merit can be made.[16]

Notes

1   "Age, Sex, Existing Conditions of COVID-19 Cases and Deaths," www.worldometers.info/coronavirus/coronavirus-age-sex-demographics.

2   "Global Recession Increases Malnutrition for the Most Vulnerable People in Developing Countries," United Nations Standing Committee on Nutrition, 2009.

3   John P.A. Ioannidis, "A Fiasco in the Making? As the Coronavirus Pandemic Takes Hold, We Are Making Decisions without Reliable Data," *STAT*, 17 March 2020.

4   "Age Structure," *The World Factbook*, Central Intelligence Agency.

5   "Global Recession Increases Malnutrition for the Most Vulnerable People in Developing Countries," United Nations Standing Committee on Nutrition, 2009.

6   "How Important Is Tourism to the South African Economy?," *Statistics South Africa*, 26 March 2018.

7   "South Africa Unemployment Rate 2000–2019 Data," *Trading Economics*, www.tradingeconomics.com.

8   "Financial Support for Businesses during Coronavirus (COVID-19)," gov.uk, 3 April 2020.

9   Kabous le Roux, "South Africans Are Drowning in Debt but Still Clamouring for Credit," *CapeTalk*, 11 October 2019.

10   Kwandokuhle Njoli, "Caprisa's Prof Karim Lauded for HIV/AIDS Efforts in Africa," *IOL*, 27 November 2018.

11   Ben Johnson, "The Great Plague 1665—the Black Death," *Historic UK*.

12   Thomas Perls, "Social Distancing: What It Is and Why It's the Best Tool We Have to Fight the Coronavirus," *The Conversation*, 13 March 2020.

13   "Age, Sex, Existing Conditions of COVID-19 Cases and Deaths," www.worldometers.info/coronavirus/coronavirus-age-sex-demographics.

14   Peter Lloyd-Sherlock, et al., "Bearing the Brunt of COVID-19: Older People in Low and Middle Income Countries," *BMJ*, 13 March 2020.

15 Alex Broadbent, "What Could Possibly Go Wrong?—A Heuristic for Predicting Population Health Outcomes of Interventions," *Preventive Medicine*, vol. 53, nos. 4–5, October–November 2011.

16 Alex Broadbent, "Thinking Rationally About Coronavirus COVID-19 (guest post by Alex Broadbent)," *Daily Nous* (blog), 9 March 2020.

CASE STUDY

Staying in Business

Jason Mullen owns and manages 5-Star Lunch and Dinner, an independent restaurant in a major urban center. 5-Star offers low-cost comfort food, served in a dining area that can accommodate 30–40 customers at small booths and tables with limited space between them. Business had been steady for over a decade, with a loyal base of regular customers and reliable tourist traffic. 5-Star operates on slim margins due to its low pricing and the substantial rent required to operate in a normally busy commercial neighborhood.

With the rapid spread of COVID-19, it was announced that restaurants state-wide would be limited to delivery and take-out only. Jason decided to temporarily close, with the expectation that business would decline to such a degree that his operating costs would outpace sales. He canceled all of his employees' scheduled shifts, offering them assurance that 5-Star would resume business once circumstances allowed.

The restaurant is Jason's sole source of income, and though far from wealthy, he expects that his own personal savings would allow him to get by for at least six months if absolutely necessary. However, the restaurant's ten regular employees—six servers and four kitchen staff—are not all as financially secure, and Jason worries about their ability to weather a lengthy closure of the restaurant. The majority of 5-Star's employees are relatively recent immigrants, and several of them financially support their spouses, children, and elderly family members. Jason worries that government support will not be enough for his employees to pay their bills, and he's bothered by the fact that the closure of restaurants and other service industry businesses is disproportionately affecting minorities and blue-collar workers.

Six weeks after closing the doors, 5-Star has increased its debt considerably in order to continue paying rent and other fixed costs. Jason expects that he can continue to pay 5-Star's expenses for another month at most but that he will soon have to either reopen or fold the business. Recent government announcements indicate that restaurants will be allowed to resume dine-in service within two weeks, provided that certain distancing measures are employed, including a maximum seating of 50 per cent of regular capacity. Jason is eager to reopen, as he expects that this is the only way to keep the business afloat. However, he worries about the potential spread of illness to both his employees and his customers.

Jason's employees have mixed feelings about returning to the job. Two of them have moved on and aren't interested in coming back. Three others feel that they must get back to work as soon as possible regardless of their apprehensions, as they'll be unable to continue paying for groceries and rent if they don't receive a paycheck soon. The other five have strong concerns about the risks of spreading infection—especially to their own families. They tell Jason that they won't be willing to return unless infection rates further decline and the risk is reduced.

What should Jason do? He knows that reopening carries the very real risk that an employee or customer could become infected despite all efforts to maintain physical distancing and sterilize surfaces. Reopening might save the restaurant, but even this is uncertain given that tourist traffic through the neighborhood will be massively reduced. On the other hand, not reopening would undoubtedly doom the business and leave both Jason and his employees jobless.

If Jason does reopen, he'll need the help of more than three staff members. Should he hire replacements for the employees who don't want to return? His stomach turns at the thought of demanding that his employees either put themselves and their families at risk or lose their jobs. Jason has heard that low-wage workers in some other industries have received raises in recognition of their essential infrastructure role. However, in contrast to grocery stores and couriers, revenue at restaurants has declined, and 5-Star's finances won't allow for employee raises at this time.

Should Jason resume operations, with the knowledge that this may put his employees at risk? He's well aware of the statistics showing how the infections and deaths due to COVID-19 have disproportionately affected ethnic minorities and low-wage workers, and he fears that reopening 5-Star will contribute to that trend; should this weigh into his decision?

Even at half capacity, the tight seating of the restaurant's dining area would require customers to be less than six feet apart from one another.

Though he's familiar with the latest guidelines on sanitation procedures, Jason worries that he and his staff lack expertise in the kinds of cleaning practices needed to minimize the risk of spreading the virus. To what degree should a business owner or manager concern themselves with public health, assuming they're following all of the mandatory guidelines?

QUESTIONS FOR REFLECTION

1. How should a health-care system or government address matters of inequity, especially in the context of a pandemic when inequities may be exacerbated? Consider the various forms of justice described in the "key terms" section of this chapter (distributive, restorative, retributive, social). Does one or another of those forms of justice best address the forms of inequality outlined by the readings in this chapter?

2. In order to satisfy domestic obligations of justice, must we have publicly funded, universal health insurance?

3. Are there global obligations of justice, or do nations have obligations of justice only to their own citizens? Do these obligations shift when in the midst of a pandemic?

6

Research Ethics

INTRODUCTION

Modern policies on the ethics of medical research were first codified in the mid- to late twentieth century in response to a number of historical abuses, perhaps most infamously the heinous experiments conducted by the Nazis during World War II. However, the history of unethical research is hardly limited to Nazi Germany; researchers in the United States and other countries likewise took advantage of vulnerable populations and engaged in conduct that would be legally prohibited today. As one of many such examples, we can look to the Tuskegee syphilis experiments performed from the 1930s to the 1970s, in which hundreds of African American men known to be infected with syphilis were neither treated nor informed of their condition while researchers studied the effects of their untreated illness.

Early guidelines for ethical research focused primarily on the protection of research participants from the dangers involved. In the 1980s, as the HIV/AIDS epidemic spread, the range of ethical concerns was broadened. HIV patients began to ask for access to new medications that were still being tested, knowing that without these experimental drugs they might not survive until fully tested and approved treatments became widely available. At that time, many countries developed what are sometimes known as "right to try" laws allowing the compassionate use of medicines that had not yet been approved for use outside of clinical trials.

It should be remembered, however, that providing patients with drugs that have not been fully tested is a dangerous practice. We conduct research precisely when we do not know whether a drug, vaccine, or treatment will be safe and effective in humans, and there are countless examples of trials in which initially promising treatments turned out to be dangerous—in some cases, more dangerous than the underlying conditions they were intended to treat.

Current research ethics policies attempt to strike a delicate balance between protecting participants and providing access to urgently needed medications for novel diseases. During a pandemic, this balance is particularly tricky, as there is significant social and political pressure to accelerate ordinary research practices and to permit treatments that haven't yet undergone standard trials. This chapter examines several arguments and proposals as to how the balance should be achieved.

In the first reading, Julian Savulescu lays out the issues involved in deciding how to ethically design a trial for COVID-19 treatments and vaccines. He notes that, although the standards of research ethics should be upheld, any delay in finding a treatment or vaccine will cost human lives.

Nir Eyal, Marc Lipsitch, and Peter G. Smith argue in favor of randomized, double-anonymized, placebo-controlled human challenge studies. Their proposal involves randomly sorting research participants into a vaccinated group and a placebo group. Neither the researchers nor the participants will know which group they are in (i.e., whether they received the vaccine or saline water). All participants would then be infected with SARS-CoV-2. Eyal et al. argue that, with a number of safety measures in place and with the informed consent of all research participants, the risks of such a trial would be outweighed by the tremendous potential benefits of a vaccine.

Human challenge studies, in which participants are deliberately infected with a disease, are controversial. They generate results much faster than standard vaccine trials, in which researchers inject vaccinations and then simply wait to see whether participants become infected through ordinary day-to-day life. For one thing, the vaccine used in a human challenge study might not confer any protection at all. Furthermore, in a human challenge study such as the one proposed by Eyal et al., only some of the research participants will receive the vaccine; the other half will be infected with the virus without receiving a vaccination. Is informed and autonomous consent sufficient to authorize these risks? People do seem willing to take part in such trials. As of 22 April 2020, around 1,500 people had signed up to participate in a vaccine challenge study, even though none had yet been approved.[1] But are those who sign up for challenge studies doing so in an informed way, or are they potentially basing their decisions on false hope?

In the next reading of this section, Kelly McBride Folkers and Arthur Caplan caution that people may have mistaken ideas about the probable benefits of COVID-19 treatments and potential vaccines. We are inundated daily with articles, press conferences, and television news programs that report on allegedly promising preliminary data from clinical trials. In the end, some of these have turned out to be based more on hype and hope than on fact.

KEY TERMS

active controlled trial: a clinical trial in which the control group receives the standard of care (i.e., the best-known treatment for the condition in question) rather than a placebo. Active controlled trials have fewer risks for the subjects but take longer to yield results. Active controlled trials are preferred when there is a known treatment for a condition.

anonymized trial: a trial in which either the researcher or the subject is not aware which group the subject is in. (Previously called "blinded" trials, although this terminology is outdated and has ableist assumptions.)

challenge study: a trial in which research subjects are deliberately infected with a live virus to determine the effectiveness of a vaccine or intervention. The advantage of challenge studies is that they may yield results more quickly than standard trial protocols. The disadvantage is that they place research subjects at considerable risks. If a challenge study is placebo controlled, then some research subjects will be exposed to the virus without receiving any protection.

clinical trial: a research study using human subjects that aims to test the effects of a medical intervention.

double-anonymized trial: a trial in which neither the researcher nor the subject knows which group the subject is in.

placebo: a substance that has no therapeutic effect, such as a sugar pill or a saline injection.

placebo-controlled trial: a clinical trial in which the control group receives no intervention. Placebos, such as sugar pills or saline injections, are often used so that the researcher and subjects do not know which subjects are receiving intervention and which subjects are in the control group.

randomized trial: a research study in which the subjects are randomly allocated to one group (e.g., placebo arm) or the other (e.g., active arm).

NOTE

1 Ewen Callaway, "Hundreds of People Volunteer to Be Infected with Coronavirus," *Nature*, 22 April 2020, https://www.nature.com/articles/d41586-020-01179-x.

6.1

Is It Right to Cut Corners in the Search for a Coronavirus Cure?

Julian Savulescu

Vaccine and drug trials are slow, to account for safety. But in a pandemic time isn't just money—it's lives.

The race is on to find a treatment for coronavirus. This race is split between two approaches: the trialling of pre-existing drugs used for similar diseases, and the hunt for a vaccine. In both instances, important ethical decisions must be made. Is it OK to reassign a treatment that comes with side-effects? And with thousands dying from coronavirus every day, is it acceptable to cut corners in the search for a vaccine?

Last Friday [20 March, 2020], the World Health Organization announced the launch of Solidarity, a worldwide trial of the four most promising candidate treatments for COVID-19: remdesivir, an antiretroviral treatment for Ebola; chloroquine and hydroxychloroquine, both antimalarials; ritonavir, an HIV treatment; and interferon, a treatment for hepatitis C. Both Kaiser Permanente Washington Research Institute in Seattle and China's Academy of Military Medical Sciences last week announced the start of human trials for new possible vaccines. Around 30 other research groups worldwide are working on vaccines.

But the WHO estimates that a vaccine won't be ready until June 2021. There are requirements that have to be observed. The gold standard for this kind of research is the clinical trial—administering the vaccine to a large number of people in controlled conditions and measuring its effect. Usually scientists wait 14 months to monitor effectiveness and possible side-effects—which is why we may have to wait until next summer. Coronavirus vaccine trials face the following dilemma: we need treatment quickly but we also need to know it will work. The worst outcome for the medical industry would be a vaccine that either did not work or, worse, was harmful or had side-effects. Globally, faith in vaccines is already at an all-time low.

Decisions are taken by governments, in tandem with ethics committees. Every day they delay the development or introduction of an intervention found to be effective, a growing number will die. There have so far been 19,603 deaths, with 12% of those deaths occurring in a single day—yesterday (Tuesday 24 March).

The economic devastation being wrought must also be considered—this will cost lives through depression, suicide and other effects of deprivation. In a pandemic, time is not only money. It is lives. Many lives.

Yet even promising possible treatments can prove to be ineffective or even harmful. Remdesivir, chloroquine, ritonavir and interferon all have serious side-effects, including heart arrhythmias and possibly death. Indeed, a man in Arizona died after ingesting chloroquine, believing it would protect him from COVID-19.

In terms of vaccine discovery, there are plenty of ways authorities could speed up the process. One is a human challenge study. This involves deliberately infecting a person with coronavirus to look at how the virus behaves and using that evidence to find the most promising vaccines. Today, healthy people are deliberately infected with flu, common cold, typhoid, malaria, dengue fever and streptococcal infections to study the disease, and more rapidly develop vaccines and treatments.

Challenge studies have been proposed in COVID-19. Hvivo, a clinical research group in London, has attracted more than 20,000 volunteers willing to be infected with a milder coronavirus that does not cause serious symptoms. They will each be paid £3,500. However, the utility of studying a related virus may be limited. There have been suggestions of challenge studies infecting younger participants at lower risk of complication with COVID-19. This comes with dangers and profound ethical implications—but could save thousands of lives. Another alternative would be to conscript low-risk people likely to be exposed to COVID-19 anyway to vaccine trials. A benefit of this would be to accrue a large sample group, so helping to indicate whether treatments could be rolled out to large populations. It is notable that China's vaccine testing will occur within a military installation: the suggestion is that trials may be conducted on soldiers without consent.

This war will require lines to be drawn: what level of uncertainty to accept, whether research can be done on unconscious patients without consent, what level of risk is justifiable, and so on. Currently these decisions are usually made by ethics committees using guidelines developed for non-pandemic situations. We require leadership from the government to push ahead scientific research around all treatment options, while ensuring reasonable risks. In my opinion, a failure by government to support this research is as wrong as implementing harmful policy.

How quickly we develop a treatment or a cure will depend on the risks we are prepared to take. So far, western countries have given greater priority to liberty and rights than eastern countries in responding to coronavirus, leaving them less able to secure public health. It is now, most likely, too late to eliminate the virus with isolation and quarantine. Scientific research looks the most promising option for a resolution to this pandemic.

We need to run the race by the rules in order to sufficiently protect human participants. But there is a balance to be struck: let's not run it with one hand tied behind our back.

6.2

Human Challenge Studies to Accelerate Coronavirus Vaccine Licensure

Nir Eyal, Marc Lipsitch, and Peter G. Smith

Alleviation of the enormous burden of mortality and morbidity associated with the COVID-19 pandemic will probably depend on the development of effective vaccines that could be rolled out widely. Many candidate vaccines are in development,[1] but recent estimates cite at least 1–1.5 years to vaccine rollout.[2] A significant proportion of that time is due to the requirement to assess efficacy and safety in placebo-controlled Phase 3 trials, which typically involve several thousand participants followed for long enough in the field to assess differences in disease incidence between vaccine and control groups, with many participants taking precautions to avoid exposure. We suggest that, in the circumstances of a devastating global pandemic, controlled human challenge studies (following the normal initial safety, vaccine dose finding, and immunogenicity studies—phases 1/2 in Figure 1) may be an acceptable way to bypass Phase 3 testing, and speed the licensure of efficacious vaccines.

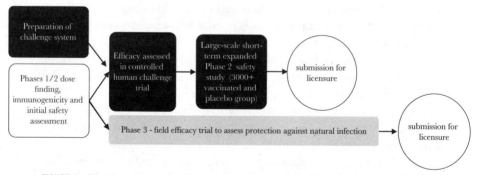

FIGURE 1 The process to vaccine licensure through a controlled human challenge trial and large study to assess short-term safety (black); compared to the conventional Phase 3 trial route to licensure (grey). Submission for licensure could occur substantially earlier with a controlled human challenge trial.

The Proposed Study Design

Volunteers for human challenge studies would be drawn from previously uninfected individuals at relatively low risk of complications or mortality from SARS-CoV-2 infection (e.g. young adults, without chronic health conditions and not otherwise sick)[3-7] and who are at substantial risk of natural exposure to SARS-CoV-2 (e.g. resident in areas with high transmission rates). Such a target group might comprise uninfected persons aged 20–45 years, an age range in which the risk of death or serious complications following infection is substantially lower than in older age groups.[4,5]

The controlled challenge model would need to be standardized before using it to test vaccines. Volunteers, previously uninfected, would be required for an initial dose-escalation study of the viral challenge to select a dose of virus exposure such that most placebo recipients become infected (for statistical reasons), and have a clinical response that is not more severe than the one associated with natural infection (for ethical reasons). The latter would require comparison with a cohort of individuals of similar age who had been infected naturally. For this standardization, volunteers may spend two weeks in a clinical isolation facility prior to the challenge, with viral and serologic testing, to exclude those with previous or recent infection (or a shorter duration if suitable serological tests for recent infections are developed). Overall, these preparatory studies (upper-left black square in Figure 1) may take several weeks, and could start before vaccine candidates are available for evaluation.

Multiple measures would be put in place to ensure that prior to consenting, potential participants fully comprehend the unusual risks involved in the study.

After the controlled human challenge model had been set up, vaccines could be evaluated. Volunteers who had not been previously infected would be randomized to receive either the candidate vaccine(s) under investigation, or placebo. After an interval to permit a full immune response to the vaccine, a controlled exposure to SARS-CoV-2 would be administered. Appropriate vaccine schedules (e.g. dose, number of doses) will have been determined, to the extent possible, in the conventional Phase 1/2 immunogenicity and safety studies that preceded the challenge study.

Following the challenge, the participants would be carefully followed, to monitor whether those vaccinated had a different response to viral challenge. Because the challenge studies would be relatively small and some volunteers might show few clinical symptoms, there would need to be careful consideration of the choice of the primary endpoint, through discussions with regulatory authorities. Possibilities would include viral load, measured at least daily (e.g. in throat swabs), and then cumulated over the course of the infection (as has been done in influenza challenge studies),[8] and time to first clinical symptoms. For some vaccines, the endpoint might be the proportion infected. Throughout the study, intense immunological monitoring would seek any correlates of vaccine effect. The required size of such studies would depend upon the endpoints chosen, but they might require of the order of 100 volunteers.

Any volunteers in whom infection was confirmed would receive excellent care for COVID-19, including priority for any scarce life-saving resources, in state-of-the-art facilities. Throughout the trial and until infectiousness were ruled out, all participants would remain isolated in a secure and comfortable setting.

If this human challenge study showed a vaccine candidate to be efficacious, an expanded placebo-controlled study would be conducted in the field, involving at least 3000 vaccinated persons, primarily for short-term safety assessment, but also to gather further evidence on immunogenicity (in Figure 1, right-most black box). Participants would be carefully monitored for adverse effects following vaccination, to gather safety data sufficient for submission for licensure. This study (not involving a challenge) should be conducted on the eventual primary initial target group for an effective vaccine—including the elderly and those with concomitant illnesses that increase the risk of serious disease following infection. With prior planning, this large-scale assessment of safety could be completed in several months, as initially only short-term adverse effects would be assessed.

Together, the information from the challenge study and the short-term follow-up of those in the expanded (Phase 2) field study may produce evidence sufficient to justify accelerated licensure.

Participants of the expanded field study could continue to be followed longer term in parallel with the submission for licensure, so that suitable actions could be taken if any long-term adverse effects, including disease enhancement, were identified. As with standard vaccine licensure, additional, post-approval studies would be required to assess safety and effectiveness in routine use. Any necessary studies of dosage and safety in special groups (e.g. children, pregnant women, immuno-compromised) could be conducted, before extending vaccination to these groups, if judged appropriate.

It is possible that the protection that was apparent in a challenge study will not be replicated when the vaccine is used to protect against natural infection. This would have to be carefully monitored in the early stages of vaccine rollout, for example through case-control studies. In such an event, appropriate modification will be made to the vaccination program (including potentially stopping vaccination).

A particular concern with respect to some vaccine constructs against coronavirus is that they may induce more severe disease following infection, as has been reported in animal models of both SARS and MERS vaccine candidates[9] If any vaccine candidate shows evidence of such effects in animal models, it is likely to be ruled out for human testing. However, for those candidates that are taken forward for human testing, the possibility of enhancement should be borne in mind and the challenge studies should be designed in such a way that small groups of volunteers are challenged sequentially. This way, studies could be stopped at an early stage, upon first strong indication of vaccine-induced enhanced disease. If the vaccine candidate did enhance disease, the controlled human challenge model would provide much more rapid evidence to support stopping the testing of a harmful vaccine candidate, with far fewer vaccinated persons, than a traditional Phase 3 efficacy study.

Acceleration of Licensure, and Substantial Social Value

The proposed trial method would potentially cut the wait time for the rollout of an efficacious vaccine. Challenge studies (which always directly expose all participants to a pathogen to assess efficacy) generally require fewer participants, followed over a shorter period than do standard efficacy studies (in which many participants are never exposed). Rollout of an efficacious vaccine to age groups not included in the challenge studies may depend on immunological bridging, but this would be a component of the expanded safety studies discussed above. It is possible that this process could take several months shorter than reliance on standard Phase 3 testing to assess efficacy. While rollout to other populations might require initial bridging studies, these could be conducted relatively quickly.

It seems clear that, in the absence of an efficacious vaccine, hundreds of thousands of persons globally are going to die prematurely from COVID-19. Intense social distancing and related control measures, held in place for many months between now and the availability of vaccine, will themselves take a toll on economies, societies, and population health. Advancing the registration and rollout of an efficacious vaccine, even by a few months, could save many thousands of lives and commands enormous societal value.

Autonomous Authorization

Deliberate exposure of study participants to SARS-CoV-2 clearly raises ethical concerns. It may seem impermissible to ask people to take on risk of severe illness or death, even for an important collective gain. But we actually ask people to take such risks for others' direct gain every time we ask volunteer firefighters to rush into burning buildings; relatives to donate a live organ to loved ones; healthy volunteers to participate in drug and vaccine toxicity trials with no prospect of improving their health (and some risk of undermining it);[10] relatively healthy volunteers to participate in studies involving long antiretroviral drug interruptions that risk their health with negligible prospect of improving it,[11] and other challenge studies in which healthy volunteers expose themselves to pathogens.[12] This spring, we are clearly within our right when we invite citizens to volunteer for Emergency Medical Services (EMS) to fight a pandemic that augments both the personal risks for EMS workers and the social value of their work; and initial trials for the Moderna SARS-CoV-2 vaccine are being accelerated by skipping prior animal testing and the margin of safety that it would have added.[13]

One major reason why it is permissible to risk medical harm to volunteers in medical studies, even when their personal healthcare does not require that risk, is that these volunteers will have autonomously consented to take on these risks. Adult persons can legitimize many interventions in their bodies and health that are normally prohibited, simply by saying "Yes", with full understanding and voluntariness. In the present case, the study would involve multiple tests of comprehension of all risks, so that the decision is deeply informed and voluntary. The exclusive recruitment of participants older than 20 years, although children are less likely to have severe symptoms upon COVID-19 infection,[6, 7] seeks to safeguard the quality of participants' consent. The wide news coverage and widespread fear of COVID-19 should keep it clear that exposure to this virus is no small matter. While in other studies mentioned above, non-consenting sex partners and fetuses of study participants may get infected,[14, 15] the proposed controlled challenge study would avoid risk to non-participants by isolating participants whilst infectious.

Added Risk Remains Acceptable

But a remaining key question, for deeming human challenge studies ethical, pertains to risk. Are the risks to participants, even when they are justified by the social importance of the trial and backed by participants' willful permission, also being kept to the necessary minimum? And do the risks fall below a postulated cap on the acceptable risk of medical trials, even ones of the highest social value and with participants' consent?[14]

The proposed challenge studies seek to contain the risk to participants in five different ways. First, the study will recruit only healthy patients from age groups in which the risk of severe disease and death following SARS-CoV-2 infection is low. Second, there is the possibility that the vaccine candidate will protect at least some of those who are vaccinated. Third, in the absence of an effective vaccine, a high proportion of the general population is likely to be naturally infected with SARS-CoV-2 at some point,[16] including those who might participate in a challenge study; by volunteering to be artificially infected they may be just hastening an event that is likely to occur in later months anyhow. Fourth, only people with an especially high baseline risk of getting exposed during or soon after the trial period should be recruited, e.g. people residing in areas with high transmission rates. Fifth, participants would be monitored carefully and frequently following the challenge, and afforded the best available care if needed, e.g. guaranteed access to state of the art facilities of the health system, notwithstanding the possibility of severe shortages of medical care during the evolving pandemic. For these five reasons, mortality and morbidity from participation notwithstanding, *net* mortality and morbidity from participation should remain low, or negative.

Conclusion

A novel strain of Coronavirus forces us to consider unconventional approaches. We believe that controlled SARS-CoV-2 vaccine challenge studies may accelerate the time it takes to evaluate and license vaccines and hence could make vaccines available sooner for widespread rollout.

Such an approach is not without risks, but every week that vaccine rollout is delayed will be accompanied by many thousands of deaths globally. Importantly, challenge studies are conducted against the background of competent volunteers' informed consent, minimization of study risks, and high baseline risks of infection for participants. They do not violate participants' individual rights on the altar of emergency response, but heed both individual rights and the global public health emergency.

References

1 WHO. DRAFT landscape of COVID-19 candidate vaccines. Available at: https://www.who.int/blueprint/priority-diseases/key-action/novel-coronavirus-landscape-ncov.pdf?ua=1. Accessed March 20 2020.

2 Spinney L. When will a coronavirus vaccine be ready? Guardian, 2020.

3 CDC. People at Risk for Serious Illness from COVID-19. Available at: https://www.cdc.gov/coronavirus/2019-ncov/specific-groups/high-risk-complications.html. Accessed March 8 2020.

4 Begley S. Who is getting sick, and how sick? A breakdown of coronavirus risk by demographic factors. STATnews, 2020.

5 The Novel Coronavirus Pneumonia Emergency Response Epidemiology Team. Vital Surveillances: The Epidemiological Characteristics of an Outbreak of 2019 Novel Coronavirus Diseases (COVID-19)—China, 2020. CCDC Weekly 2020; 2:113–22.

6 Bi Q, Wu Y, Mei S, et al. Epidemiology and Transmission of COVID-19 in Shenzhen China: Analysis of 391 cases and 1,286 of their close contacts. medRxiv 2020.

7 Xu Y, Li X, Zhu B, et al. Characteristics of pediatric SARS-CoV-2 infection and potential evidence for persistent fecal viral shedding. Nature Medicine 2020.

8 Sherman AC, Mehta A, Dickert NW, Anderson EJ, Rouphael N. The Future of Flu: A Review of the Human Challenge Model and Systems Biology for Advancement of Influenza Vaccinology. Front Cell Infect Microbiol 2019; 9.

9 Wan Y, Shang J, Sun S, et al. Molecular Mechanism for Antibody-Dependent Enhancement of Coronavirus Entry. J Virol 2020; 94.

10 Miller FG. The Ethical Challenges of Human Research: Selected Essays 1st Edition. New York: Oxford UP, 2012.

11 Eyal N, Holtzman LG, Deeks S. Ethical issues in HIV remission trials. Curr Opin HIV AIDS 2018; 13.

12 Cohen J. Studies that intentionally infect people with disease-causing bugs are on the rise. Science 2016.

13 Boodman E. Researchers rush to test coronavirus vaccine in people without knowing how well it works in animals. STATnews, 2020.

14 Shah SK, Kimmelman J, Lyerly AD, et al. Ethical considerations for Zika virus human challenge trials. National Institute for Allergy and Infectious Diseases, 2017.

15 Eyal N, Deeks SG. Risk to Nonparticipants in HIV Remission Studies with Treatment Interruption: A Symposium. J Infect Dis 2019; 220:S1–S4.

16 Ferguson NM, Laydon D, Nedjati-Gilani G, et al. Impact of non-pharmaceutical interventions (NPIs) to reduce COVID-19 mortality and healthcare demand. London: Imperial College, 2020.

6.3

False Hope about Coronavirus Treatments

Kelly McBride Folkers and Arthur Caplan

While patients can and do recover from coronavirus infections, there are currently no approved treatments that are known to work against COVID-19. President Trump believes otherwise. He said at his press briefing [on 19 March 2020], that two drugs, hydroxychloroquine and remdesivir, were "essentially approved for prescribed use" to treat COVID-19 infected patients.[1] He referred to these "approvals" as a "tremendous breakthrough," and applauded Food and Drug Administration Commissioner Stephen Hahn and the agency's scientists for their quick work approving these medications. Commissioner Hahn took to the podium to clarify the president's message, saying that these drugs are not yet, in fact, known to be safe and effective treatments for coronavirus infections.

Once again, President Trump has misled the American people on the nation's response to the pandemic. In an ideal world, there would be several drugs in rich supply around the world that could be used immediately and safely to restore health to patients with severe, life-threatening coronavirus infections. However, until scientists interpret reliable data from rigorously designed studies, it is irresponsible and reckless for the country's leaders to claim that there are medicines available, just waiting to be used.

The President prattled on about one of his favorite fantasies, the importance of "right to try" legislation. For decades, the FDA has allowed physicians treating patients with severe or life-threatening illnesses, who have exhausted all approved treatment options or who cannot participate in clinical trials, to request the use of experimental drugs through a system called "compassionate use." Generally, the most common way that patients access experimental drugs is by participating in a clinical research study, in which scientists gather data on the safety and effectiveness of that drug for a particular indication, in a specific group of patients with the same health condition. There simply aren't enough spots in clinical trials for everyone who wants to participate. And some individuals may not meet a trial's strict eligibility criteria, particularly if they have multiple health conditions or are dying. But, for patients who have exhausted every other possible option, the FDA has created the compassionate use pathway for those individuals to seek access to the medical products already being tested in clinical trials.

In the context of coronavirus, this means that the FDA is working to expand access to potential therapeutic options in development. Experimental drugs or drugs already approved for other conditions that may—or may not—successfully treat coronavirus infections could, theoretically, be prescribed to patients. Hydroxychloroquine, for example, is already approved to treat malaria and certain arthritic conditions, and some experts believe it might work against COVID-19. The existing literature on the drug is not, contrary to the president, promising.

Remdesivir is different. It is an experimental antiviral drug that, according to extremely limited data in animals, may have potential activity against COVID-19. Its manufacturer, Gilead, is currently conducting randomized studies in adults diagnosed with COVID-19 in several Asian countries. Remdesivir is not yet approved anywhere in the world. For patients in the US to access either medication, they would have to enroll in a clinical trial conducted in the US or have their physician request that the drug's manufacturer make it available through compassionate use. Importantly, companies are not legally obligated to make their drugs-in-development available, for any reason, at any time. The FDA cannot make them. Nor can right to try legislation.

[As of 20 March 2020], there is no reliable data to suggest that either hydroxychloroquine or remdesivir, or any other drugs for that matter, can successfully treat COVID-19. There simply isn't enough information available yet to safely make these medicines available for widespread use. While the FDA allows patients to access drugs in development as a last resort, this is by no means a guarantee that anyone will recover. In fact, patients could get worse because of an experimental drug. Using unapproved medications in a fact-free environment will do more harm than good, possibly making a severe illness worse or even hastening death, while not allowing anyone to learn anything about what actually works.

President Trump sorely misunderstands the drug development system. But even more egregiously, he has given the nation and desperate patients false hope about what options are widely available to treat those fighting for their lives. By suggesting that these drugs are sitting on shelves just waiting to be used, the president will increase public demand for medicines that may not be safe, effective, in abundant supply or wise to use right now.

Clinical research exists for a very good reason: the vast majority of medicines that are tested in humans are not safe or effective. And even in a pandemic, carefully conducted science must rule the day to ensure that doctors are not inadvertently harming their patients by treating them with an intervention that lacks scientific evidence to support its use. Commissioner Hahn said it best: "We need to make sure that this sea of new treatments will get the right drug, to the right patient, at the right dosage, at the right time." The only way to achieve this goal is through research, not by spreading false hope about the right to try.

Note
1 Anna Edney, "Trump Touts Drug That FDA Says Isn't Yet Approved for Virus," *Bloomberg*, 19 March 2020.

CASE STUDY

Ethics and Global Research Programs

Dr. Arman Asadour is an American physician and researcher who is part of a team participating in a global SARS-CoV-2 vaccine trial. He is sent to a town in northern Nigeria near Katsina. Nigeria has had thousands of confirmed cases of COVID-19, and over 100 people have died.

Dr. Asadour spends time in the town to get to know the residents and build trust with the potential research participants. He is moved by the warmth, joy, and kindness of the townspeople, who often bring him gifts despite their poverty. They have also organized a number of citizen-powered welfare initiatives to help those who are out of work due to the pandemic.[1] However, Dr. Asadour discovers that the local infrastructure is seriously inadequate to the requirements of the research: the existing health-care resources are limited, and sanitation infrastructure is poor. In addition, there is widespread distrust toward global health organizations due to the negative perception of attempts to eradicate polio in the early 2000s. Many people in the region believe that the polio vaccines administered at that time were actually population control measures.[2]

Dr. Asadour and the research team set up an assessment tent where they will test the townspeople to determine who has COVID-19. They have a Memorandum of Understanding with the local health authority to test only the vaccine on the participants in the trial. People with other conditions and those not in the trial must be sent to the local hospital, though it is already beyond capacity.

Dr. Asadour is conscious of his ethical and legal mandate. However, he finds it difficult to refrain from administering treatment to those who don't qualify for the trial. Those who test positive for COVID-19 are to be transferred to the local hospital. But Dr. Asadour worries that the resources of the hospital may be inadequate and that sending them additional patients will result in overcrowding and added transportation and medication expenses that will put further stress on the local health system. Other potential participants in the trial have serious but treatable conditions, such as meningitis, for which the local hospital has few resources. The research team has emergency medical supplies that could save the lives of some of those people. Would it be unethical for Dr. Asadour to violate his mandate and treat such conditions, which he could do at little expense of time or resources?

Beside these clinical worries are a number of geopolitical concerns. Dr. Asadour wonders whether international clinical trials simply undermine efforts by local authorities to develop sustainable responses to COVID-19 and to improve their health care more broadly. During clinical trials, the voices and priorities of local communities are often overlooked in favor of the interests of researchers and funding agencies. And when a trial is completed or withdrawn, local service may be destabilized by the sudden absence of the research team.

Furthermore, Dr. Asadour worries that this research may contribute to a long history of exploitative and racist experimentation abroad. French researcher Dr. Jean-Paul Mira suggested that COVID-19 trials should be conducted "in Africa, where there are no masks, no treatment, no resuscitation... a bit like as it is done elsewhere for some studies on AIDS. In prostitutes, we try things because we know that they are highly exposed and that they do not protect themselves."[3] These remarks were widely and understandably criticized and Dr. Mira later apologized. Didier Drogba, a retired footballer, wrote on Twitter, "It is totally inconceivable we keep cautioning on this. Africa isn't a testing lab. I would like to vividly denounce those demeaning, false and most of all deeply racist words."[4]

How should Dr. Asadour decide what to do? Given the systemic problems with international research trials, especially in impoverished regions, should he participate at all? If he does participate, are there any special measures that he should take beyond what is legally required, in order to ensure that the research isn't exploitative?

Notes

1. Yomi Kazeem (24 April 2020), "Ordinary Nigerians Are Filling the Country's Major Social Welfare Gaps amid Coronavirus," *Quartz Africa*.
2. Hannah Hoechner (15 April 2020), "In Northern Nigeria, Distrust Jeopardises the Response to Coronavirus," *The Conversation*.
3. BBC (3 April 2020), "Coronavirus: France Racism Row over Doctors' Africa Testing Comments," *BBC News*.
4. Ibid.

QUESTIONS FOR REFLECTION

1. Does the race to create a viable vaccine for COVID-19 compromise the ethics of research? If so, should we allow such a compromise?

2. Under normal circumstances, the principle of "justice" in research requires that the group that is put at risk during research also be the group that benefits most from that research. For example, it would be unjust for members of a particular gender or racial group to be disproportionately represented in a risky clinical trial *unless* the expected results of that trial were meant to be of particular benefit to members of that group. In the research proposal presented by Eyal et al., the group that bears the risk of the research is composed of healthy people who are 20–45 years of age. Yet the research is intended to disproportionately benefit those who are not in that group—those who are above 45 years and who would be more likely to succumb to COVID-19.

   a. Is this departure from the principle of justice acceptable under pandemic conditions? If so, why?

   b. Much of the motivation behind modern research ethics stems from cases in which more vulnerable groups have been exploited to the benefit of less vulnerable groups (as in the Tuskegee syphilis experiments, for example). In the case of the challenge study proposed by Eyal et al., however, the suggestion is to experiment on less vulnerable groups to the benefit of more vulnerable groups. So do the previously developed ethical requirements still apply? To put this another way: is it morally acceptable to research on a less vulnerable group in order to benefit a more vulnerable group?

3. Is there a moral obligation for members of less vulnerable groups (such as 20–45-year-olds with no pre-existing health conditions) to volunteer for research studies such as that proposed by Eyal et al.? Is volunteering for such a study morally commendable but not required (i.e., supererogatory)?

7

Surveillance and Privacy

INTRODUCTION

Liberty, autonomy, privacy, and security are important values, as are the rights that follow from these values. However, none of these rights is unlimited. Arguably, my right to liberty does not entail my right to harm you, for example. Nor does my right to security mean that I can steal from you even when I am starving. The right to privacy, too, has a limit; if the police have reason to suspect me of a crime, they may be legally permitted to listen in on my phone calls or otherwise monitor me in ways that would normally be prohibited. These limits on rights are sometimes framed as "competing" rights that need to be balanced against one another. Other theorists argue that it is better to think of our rights as circumscribed by context and other circumstances. To paraphrase Margaret Olivia Little, I do not have a right to punch you in the nose that must be balanced by your right not to be punched in the nose. Instead, your right not to be harmed means that I simply have *no* right to punch you in the nose.[1] In this chapter, we examine the right to privacy and how it might be circumscribed or limited in the context of a pandemic.

Derek Thompson provides an overview of the various ways in which countries around the world have used apps and other technologies to assist in tracing contacts of people with COVID-19. Thompson describes both the use of GPS to track personal locations and the use of Bluetooth to track contacts. Although these approaches have allowed many countries in East Asia to successfully reduce their rates of infection, they also raise serious privacy concerns and introduce levels of surveillance that may seem totalitarian to those living in Western countries. Thompson believes this creates a dilemma. If we don't use these tracking apps, we won't be able to trace contacts as efficiently and prevent the spread of infection, but if we do use the apps, we may lose a significant degree of privacy.

In the next reading, self-described privacy activist Maciej Cegłowski makes the surprising argument that the pandemic justifies infringements on ordinary individual privacy rights. Cegłowski notes that the data harvested from our mobile phones are already being tracked and used in a variety of ways by private corporations. Allowing public health agencies to use tracking apps would not require that we give up any liberty that we have not already sacrificed. Cegłowski thinks there are opportunities in this pandemic to institute better safeguards for our data than currently exist. Legislation that enables public health surveillance could include privacy guarantees that would apply also to corporations.

Finally, Sean McDonald worries that digital tools developed during a pandemic may be repurposed for political ends. It is difficult to introduce such tools responsibly at the best of times, and these times are far from ideal. Not only are we facing a pandemic and an economic crisis, but international diplomacy is also weakened and geopolitical tensions are heightened. McDonald believes that in the heat of a disaster we may be inspired by fear to create techniques and tools of surveillance without the requisite thought, deliberation, and agreement.

KEY TERMS

contact tracing: a process by which a public health authority attempts to identify all of the individuals who have had physical contact with (or been in close proximity to) a person who has tested positive for an illness. Typically, those who have been in contact with the person are then themselves tested and quarantined—and their contacts likewise traced—in an attempt to contain the spread of infection.

flattening the curve: a public health strategy to slow the rate of infection so that hospitals do not exceed their surge capacity. This strategy may or may not lower the total number of cases. However, if those cases are spread over a longer period of time, it is hoped that hospitals will retain capacity to treat all of those who become ill, thus lowering mortality.

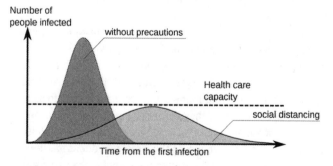

COVID-19 Health Care Limit.
Source: Image licensed under the Creative Commons Attribution-Share Alike 4.0 International license. Uploaded to commons.wikimedia.org by Johannes Kalliauer.

NOTE

1 Margaret Olivia Little (1999), "Abortion, Intimacy and the Duty to Gestate," *Ethical Theory and Moral Practice*, vol. 2, pp. 295–312.

7.1

The Technology that Could Free America from Quarantine

Derek Thompson

It's a cool fall evening in September 2020. With a bottle of wine in hand, you slide into the front seat of your car to drive to a dinner party with close friends. It's been eight months since you've seen most of them, at least outside of a computer screen.

As you're pulling out of the neighborhood, you feel your phone buzz. It's an alert from the new agency overseeing the coronavirus outbreak. On the lock screen, you can read the words "*BE ADVISED.*" Your heart sinks as you unlock the phone to read the rest of the message:

We have determined that in the past few days, you may have interacted with somebody who has recently tested positive for COVID-19. There is no need to panic. But for the sake of your family, friends, and neighbors, we are relying on your support. As soon as you can, please ...

You stop reading. You know the drill. You turn off the car, walk back into the house, and open the wine. It will be a bottle for one. Another spell of self-isolation begins now—or at least until you can get tested to prove that you don't have the coronavirus.

This could be a vision of the country's future. It is a world in which many businesses go back to normal, millions of people return to work, and social-distancing measures are relaxed, as we anxiously navigate a purgatory between the virus's early-2020 outbreak and its possible resurgence.

It is also a world in which the return to normal is predicated on the introduction of a novel technology. Millions of Americans—many of whom might be deeply skeptical of government surveillance, or Big Tech—may become participants in a national project to track their own movements and interactions, to help public-health experts map out the spread of an invisible enemy.

This is the world of "test and trace."

In the past month [i.e., since early March 2020], the coronavirus pandemic has necessitated a deep freeze of US activity. Storefronts are closed, millions of Americans have lost their jobs, and millions more are putting their health at risk in hospitals and grocery stores. This modern nightmare may not truly end until a reliable antiviral treatment or COVID-19 vaccine is widely available.

Until that day, which may be a year or two away, our best hope in the fight against the coronavirus is to play a game of sophisticated Whack-a-Mole that often goes by the name of "test and trace."

Most readers might have an image of what the testing half entails, with those long nasal swabs that practically scrape the edge of our frontal lobe. The tracing half of the equation is less understood. But it is more likely to leave its mark on American politics and society.

In its most basic form, tracing—otherwise known as tracking, or contact tracing—means identifying all the recent interactions of sick individuals to determine whom they might have infected. Testing plus tracing can besiege the virus, starve it of new bodies, and return the world to its previral routine, or something like it.

Until recently, tracing relied on an old-fashioned technology: interviews. To stop the spread of Ebola, authorities from the Centers for Disease Control and Prevention asked sick people to list recent interactions with family, friends, and businesses.[1] That interview would produce a list of contacts, who would be monitored for illness for several weeks. The state of Massachusetts recently announced plans to hire 1,000 people to do these sorts of contact-tracing interviews.[2]

But that old-school approach might not be enough. People have faulty memories about who or what they've touched, or where they've been. More important, person-to-person interviews might be too slow to arrest a national pandemic accelerating through a population.

The solution? Your phone.

Our cellphones and smartphones have several means of logging our activity. GPS tracks our location, and Bluetooth exchanges signals with nearby devices. In its most basic form, cellphone tracing might go like this: If someone tests positive for COVID-19, health officials could obtain a record of that person's cellphone activity and compare it with the data emitted by other phone owners. If officials saw any GPS overlaps (e.g., data showing that I went to a McDonald's hot spot) or Bluetooth hits (e.g., data showing that I came within several feet of a new patient), they could contact me and urge me to self-isolate, or seek a test.

Ramesh Raskar, a computer scientist at the MIT Media Lab, is working on an app that uses GPS to create maps showing the movements of people recently diagnosed with COVID-19. "In an early version, you might see a map with hot spots—2 p.m. at Starbucks, 3 p.m. at the library—that would tell you where people with the disease had recently been," Raskar told me. "All the government has to do is demand that every test facility release the trails of infected people in an anonymous manner, so that healthy people know where to avoid."

For privacy advocates, "Waze, but for the sick" might seem harvested from their darkest nightmares. But Raskar is emphatic that his code is open source— "every part of the code should be visible to everybody, every day"—and that no government or tech company would have exclusive control over a centralized database that it could abuse. Users wouldn't learn anything else about the infected person, such as age or sex.

The technology and privacy challenges of tracing will nonetheless be complex, and could normalize a level of surveillance that might seem totalitarian. If we want to get it right, we should learn from the experiences of other countries. In eastern Asia, tracing has already become a part of daily life. To see a glimpse of America's future—and to anticipate some of the worst excesses of the technology—it's useful to briefly review how tracing works across the Pacific.

Let's start with China, where citizens in hundreds of cities have been required to download cellphone software that broadcasts their location to several authorities, including the local police.[3] The app combines geotracking with other data, such as travel bookings, to designate citizens with color codes ranging from green (low risk) to red (high risk). High-risk individuals can be banned from apartment complexes, offices, and even grocery stores. Many human-rights advocates fear that what has been rolled out as a public-health app is moonlighting as a tool of government espionage and mass discrimination.[4]

Next, let's look at South Korea, a democracy that has arguably been more successful than any other in containing the spread of the virus. The government uses several sources, such as cellphone-location data, CCTV, and credit-card records, to broadly monitor citizens' activity. When somebody tests positive, local governments can send out an alert, a bit like a flood warning, that reportedly includes the individual's last name, sex, age, district of residence, and credit-card history, with a minute-to-minute record of their comings and goings from various local businesses.[5] "In some districts, public information includes which rooms of a building the person was in, when they visited a toilet, and whether or not they wore a mask," Mark Zastrow, a reporter for *Nature*, wrote. "Even overnight stays at 'love motels' have been noted."[6]

New cases in South Korea have declined about 90 percent in the past 40 days, an extraordinary achievement. But the amount of information in South Korea's tracing alerts has turned some of its citizens into imperious armchair detectives, who scour the internet in an attempt to identify people who test positive and condemn them online. Choi Young-ae, the chair of South Korea's Human Rights Commission, has said that this harassment has made some Koreans less willing to be tested.

Singapore offers perhaps the most likely model for the West. Residents can download an app called TraceTogether, which uses Bluetooth technology to keep a log of nearby devices. If somebody gets sick, that user can upload relevant data to the Ministry of Health, which notifies the owners of all the devices pinged by the infected person's phone.

"Bluetooth is much better than GPS at tracking actual contacts, and it gives a good picture of which phones come close to each other," says Ulf Buermeyer, a privacy advocate, an officer at the Berlin Department of Justice, and the president of Germany's Society for Civil Rights. "The downside of Singapore's app is that you have to register with your phone number. When a person is found infected with the disease, the authorities can easily match the IDs with associated home numbers and impose restrictive measures directly on these people."

Germany, which is helping to lead Europe's tracing efforts, is looking to tweak the Singaporean model in a way that might make it more amenable to Western sensibilities.[7] Buermeyer told me that one possibility is to program phones to broadcast a different ID every 30 minutes. So, for example, if I went to Starbucks in the morning, my phone would broadcast one ID over Bluetooth to all the other phones in the café. An hour later, at lunch with a friend, it would broadcast a different ID to all the other phones at the restaurant. Throughout the day, my phone would also receive and save IDs and log them in an encrypted Rolodex.

Days later, if I were diagnosed with the coronavirus, my doctor would ask me to upload my app's data to a central server. That server would go through my encrypted Rolodex and find all of the temporary IDs I had collected. An algorithm would match the temporary IDs to something called a push token—a unique code that connects each phone to the app. It could then send each phone an automated message through the app: *PLEASE BE ADVISED: We have determined that in the past few days, you may have interacted with somebody*... At no point in this entire process would anybody's identity be known to either the government or the tech companies operating the central server.

This brief global tour of tracing technology provides at least three lessons.

First, test and trace seems to work—period. Singapore and South Korea are very different countries from each other and from the US. But they have learned from previous outbreaks. Through tracing, both countries have reduced COVID-19 deaths much more successfully than many similarly dense US cities.

Second, the sheer amount of information made available by tracing apps will be tantalizing for power-hungry governments and data-hungry corporations to monopolize. A tracing app made necessary by the pandemic cannot become an indefinite surveillance system run by some occult government agency.

Third, the virus creates a dilemma of data. At the moment, what we don't know—who is infected, and where they have been—can kill us. Test and trace offers a road out of ignorance. But the more we seek to learn about the sick, their locations, and their contacts, the more we begin to infringe on the privacy of patients and businesses.

For the past few years, privacy advocates have criticized advertising giants such as Google and Facebook for following us around the web and harvesting our data to anticipate future behavior. Whether you found these critiques compelling or overwrought, the accusations certainly apply to tracing technology. It is easy, then, to imagine how some test-and-trace apps might be tarred as "swabs and surveillance" and rejected outright.

But while online advertising technology might mislead consumers about the nature of the task at hand, the aim of smartphone tracing is straightforward: *This is software to tell you whether your cellphone signal or daily routine intersects with a viral contagion that is killing people and destroying the economy.*

The pandemic has already required Americans to embrace extreme behavior in the name of saving lives. Tens of millions of Americans are living under house arrest. Many chief executives and entrepreneurs have said they agree with a government mandate to shut down their businesses. In these strange times, common rights that once seemed nonnegotiable have been suddenly renegotiated. Compared with our life just six weeks ago, smartphone tracing might seem like a violation of our dignity and privacy—and compared with our life six years from now, I hope it will be. But compared with our present nightmare, strategically sacrificing our privacy might be the best way to protect other freedoms.

"I am a privacy advocate, but I don't hold privacy as an absolute value," Buermeyer told me. "Privacy has to be balanced in context with other human rights. Life and health, I think, are important human rights."

Notes

1 US Department of Health and Human Services: Centers for Disease Control and Prevention, "What Is Contact Tracing?," 12 January 2016.
2 Martha Bebinger, "Why Charlie Baker Thinks 'Contact Tracing' Cases May Help Mass. Slow—Or Stop—COVID-19," *WBUR*, 3 April 2020.
3 Paul Mozur, Raymond Zhong, and Aaron Krolik, "In Coronavirus Fight, China Gives Citizens a Color Code, With Red Flags," *New York Times*, 1 March 2020.
4 Ibid.
5 Victoria Kim, Twitter post, 24 March 2020, 2:47 a.m., https://twitter.com/vicjkim/status/1242372488606052355.
6 Mark Zastrow, "South Korea Is Reporting Intimate Details of COVID-19 Cases: Has It Helped?," *Nature*, 18 March 2020.
7 Douglas Busvine, "Germany Aims to Launch Singapore-style Coronavirus App in Weeks," *Reuters*, 30 March 2020.

7.2

We Need a Massive Surveillance Program

Maciej Cegłowski

I am a privacy activist who has been riding a variety of high horses about the dangers of permanent, ubiquitous data collection since 2012.

But warning people about these dangers today is like being concerned about black mold growing in the basement when the house is on fire. Yes, in the long run the elevated humidity poses a structural risk that may make the house uninhabitable, or at least a place no one wants to live. But right now, the house is on fire. We need to pour water on it.

In our case, the fire is the global pandemic and the severe economic crisis it has precipitated. Once the initial shock wears off, we can expect this to be followed by a political crisis, in which our society will fracture along pre-existing lines of contention.

But for the moment, we are united by fear and have some latitude to act.

Doctors tell us that if we do nothing, the coronavirus will infect a large fraction of humanity over the next few months. As it spreads, the small proportion of severe cases will overwhelm the medical system, a process we are seeing play out right now in places like Lombardy and New York City. It is imperative that we slow this process down (the famous "flattening the curve") so that the peak of infections never exceeds our capacity to treat the severely ill. In the short term this can only be done by shutting down large sections of the economy, an unprecedented move.

But once the initial outbreak is contained, we will face a dilemma. Do we hurt people by allowing the economy to collapse entirely, or do we hurt people by letting the virus spread again? How do we reconcile the two?

One way out of the dilemma would be some kind of medical advance—a vaccine, or an effective antiviral treatment that lowered the burden on hospitals. But it is not clear how long the research programs searching for these breakthroughs will take, or whether they will succeed at all.

Without these medical advances, we know the virus will resume its spread as soon as the harsh controls are lifted.

Doctors and epidemiologists caution us that the only way to go back to some semblance of normality after the initial outbreak has been brought under control will be to move from population-wide measures (like closing schools and making everyone stay home) to an aggressive case-by-case approach that involves a combination of extensive testing, rapid response, and containing clusters of infection as soon as they are found, before they have a chance to spread.

That kind of case tracking has traditionally been very labor intensive. But we could automate large parts of it with the technical infrastructure of the surveillance economy. It would not take a great deal to turn the ubiquitous tracking tools that follow us around online into a sophisticated public health alert system.

Every one of us now carries a mobile tracking device that leaves a permanent trail of location data. This data is individually identifiable, precise to within a few meters, and is harvested by a remarkable variety of devices and corporations, including the large tech companies, internet service providers, handset manufacturers, mobile companies, retail stores, and in one infamous case, public trash cans on a London street.[1]

Anyone who has this data can retroactively reconstruct the movements of a person of interest, and track who they have been in proximity to over the past several days. Such a data set, combined with aggressive testing, offers the potential to trace entire chains of transmission in real time, and give early warning to those at highest risk.

This surveillance sounds like dystopian fantasy, but it exists today, ready for use. All of the necessary data is being collected and stored already. The only thing missing is a collective effort to pool it and make it available to public health authorities, along with a mechanism to bypass the few Federal privacy laws that prevent the government from looking at the kind of data the private sector can collect without restraint.

We've already seen such an ad-hoc redeployment of surveillance networks in Israel, where an existing domestic intelligence network was used to notify people that they had possibly been infected, and should self-quarantine, a message that was delivered by text message with no prior warning that such a system even existed.[2]

We could make similar quick changes to the surveillance infrastructure in the United States (hopefully with a little more public awareness that such a system was coming online). When people are found to be sick, their location and contact history could then be walked back to create a list of those they were in touch with during the period of infectiousness. Those people would then be notified of the need to self-quarantine (or hunted with blowguns and tranquilizer darts, sent to FEMA labor camps, or whatever the effective intervention turns out to be.)

This tracking infrastructure could also be used to enforce self-quarantine, using the same location-aware devices. The possibilities of such a system are many, even before you start writing custom apps for it, and there would be no shortage of tech volunteers to make it a reality.

The aggregate data set this surveillance project would generate would have enormous value in its own right. It would give public health authorities a way to identify hot spots, run experiments, and find interventions that offered the maximum benefit at the lowest social cost. They could use real-time data and projections to allocate scarce resources to hospitals, and give advance warnings of larger outbreaks to state and Federal authorities in time to inform policy decisions.

Of course, all of this would come at an enormous cost to our privacy. This is usually the point in an essay where I'd break out the old Ben Franklin quote: "those who would give up essential liberty to purchase a little temporary safety deserve neither."

But this proposal doesn't require us to give up any liberty that we didn't already sacrifice long ago, on the altar of convenience. The terrifying surveillance infrastructure this project requires exists and is maintained in good working order in the hands of private industry, where it is entirely unregulated and is currently being used to try to sell people skin cream. Why not use it to save lives?

The most troubling change this project entails is giving access to sensitive location data across the entire population to a government agency. Of course that is scary, especially given the track record of the Trump administration. The data collection would also need to be coercive (that is, no one should be able to opt out of it, short of refusing to carry a cell phone). As with any government surveillance program, there would be the danger of a ratchet effect, where what is intended as an emergency measure becomes the permanent state of affairs, like happened in the United States in the wake of the 2001 terrorist attacks.

But the public health potential of commandeering surveillance advertising is so great that we can't dismiss it out of hand. I am a privacy activist, typing this through gritted teeth, but I am also a human being like you, watching a global calamity unfold around us. What is the point of building this surveillance architecture if we can't use it to save lives in a scary emergency like this one?

One existing effort we could look to as a model for navigating this situation is the public/private partnership we have set up to monitor child sexual abuse material (CSAM) on the Internet.

Large image sharing sites like Facebook, Google, and Snapchat use a technology called PhotoDNA to fingerprint and identify images of known abuse material. They do this voluntarily, but if they find something, they are required by law to report it to the National Center for Missing and Exploited Children, a nongovernmental entity that makes referrals as appropriate to the FBI.

The system is not perfect, and right now is being used as a political football in a Trump administration attempt to curtail end-to-end encryption. But it shows the kind of public-private partnership you can duct tape together when the stakes are high and every party involved feels the moral imperative to act.

In this spirit, I believe the major players in the online tracking space should team up with the CDC, FEMA, or some other Federal agency that has a narrow remit around public health, and build a national tracking database that will operate for some fixed amount of time, with the sole purpose of containing the coronavirus epidemic. It will be necessary to pass legislation to loosen medical privacy laws and indemnify participating companies from privacy lawsuits, as well as override California's privacy law, to collect this data. I don't believe the legal obstacles are insuperable, but I welcome correction on this point by people who know the relevant law.

This enabling legislation, however, should come at a price. We have an opportunity to lay a foundation for the world we want to live in after the crisis is over. One reason we tolerate the fire department knocking down our door when there is an emergency is that we have strong protections against such intrusions, whether by government agencies or private persons, in more normal times. Those protections don't exist right now for online privacy. One reason this proposal is so easy to float is that private companies have enjoyed an outrageous freedom to track every aspect of our lives, keeping the data in perpetuity, and have made full use of it, turning the online economy into an extractive industry. That has to end.

Including privacy guarantees in the enabling legislation for public health surveillance will also help ensure that emergency measures don't become the new normal. If we use this capability deftly, we could come out of this crisis with a relatively intact economy, a low cumulative death toll, and a much healthier online sphere.

Of course, the worst people are in power right now, and the chances of them putting such a program through in any acceptable form are low. But it's 2020. Weirder things have happened. The alternative is to keep this surveillance infrastructure in place to sell soap and political ads, but refuse to bring it to bear in a situation where it can save millions of lives. That would be a shameful, disgraceful legacy indeed.

I continue to believe that living in a surveillance society is incompatible in the long term with liberty. But a prerequisite of liberty is physical safety. If temporarily conscripting surveillance capitalism as a public health measure offers us a way out of this crisis, then we should take it, and make full use of it. At the same time, we should reflect on why such a powerful surveillance tool was instantly at hand in this crisis, and what its continuing existence means for our long-term future as a free people.

Notes

1 Dan Goodin, "No, This Isn't a Scene from Minority Report. This Trash Can Is Stalking You," *Ars Technica*, 9 August 2013.

2 Daniel Estrin, "Israel Begins Tracking and Texting Those Possibly Exposed to the Coronavirus," *NPR*, 19 March 2020.

7.3

Coronavirus
A Digital Governance Emergency of International Concern

Sean McDonald

The outbreak of COVID-19 in China's Hubei province has been called a lot of things: a public health emergency of international concern, an "infodemic" and an era-defining test of the Chinese government's leadership.[1] Of course, all of those things are true. But the outbreak also sheds light on something else that's drawn much less attention so far: the extent of state power in digital spaces.

In February, in an uncommon move against the international press, the Chinese government expelled three *Wall Street Journal* reporters, ostensibly as a reaction to the paper's publication of a controversial opinion piece focusing on China's response to the emergence of the 2019 coronavirus, which causes COVID-19.[2] The journalists had nothing to do with the piece, but the incident was notable as an unusually disproportionate measure to control a foreign media outlet.

The day before the ousting, the United States announced a new policy position treating Chinese state journalists as official representatives of the Chinese state and intelligence apparatus, which is similarly unusual.[3] Earlier in the week, the United States brought criminal racketeering charges against Huawei, a partially state-owned telecommunications infrastructure and services provider.[4] The week before, over the objection of experts,[5] the US government introduced a range of travel security procedures and bans, ostensibly aimed at helping contain the COVID-19 virus—despite doing very little testing for the disease at home.[6]

Concerningly, the use of such adversarial tactics comes at a time when the United States' diplomatic corps and capacity are at historic lows—having eliminated the positions that oversee epidemic response, and appointed Vice President Mike Pence as the lead of the American efforts. In and of themselves, these tensions are remarkable, but they also frame the ways in which the world's most powerful governments respond to a global pandemic.

Epidemic response is a rare circumstance in which governments make sweeping decisions about the collective good and take unchecked action, often in contravention of individual human rights. In times of emergency, governments limit freedom of movement, seize and monitor privately collected data, and expedite the development of treatments and vaccines. In democratic societies, those powers are typically held in check by the legislature or law enforcement—but in almost all cases, those powers are exerted domestically. The growing emergence of far-reaching international epidemics poses a range of coordination challenges, many of which are complicated by negotiations over state power and access.

The global influence of technology and the abundance of personal data are already changing the balance of power between governments and citizens. In 2015, the Government of South Korea contained an outbreak of Middle East Respiratory Syndrome (MERS) by quarantining 17,000 people—in part, on the basis of their seized mobile phone records.[7] During the West African outbreak of Ebola, international response organizations helped set up national, real-time mobile surveillance systems in several of the most affected countries.[8]

And, these kinds of exercises are also being deployed to contain COVID-19. Early on, in order to find a suspected carrier of the COVID-19 virus, the United States used Uber records to track the patient to Mexico, which then caused the company to block another 240 drivers.[9] Recently, US President Donald Trump called COVID-19 a "hoax," perpetuated by his political opponents, before walking the remarks back.[10] Similarly, Taiwan's foreign minister accused the Chinese government of waging "cyber war" in order to effect its COVID-19 response.[11] Even if there was uniform agreement that these digital exertions of power were effective—and there isn't—there are very few mechanisms to articulate, check or challenge the digital limits of state power during a time of crisis.

That's concerning enough as a domestic policy issue, especially amid the growth of digital surveillance technologies, but it's even more concerning in the middle of a global health crisis. With at least 67 countries reporting cases of the virus [by 2 March 2020], that's 67 governments managing a public health emergency, generating and consuming data in varying ways about the disease, and trying to consider the growing (and fragmented) global response. The logistical undertaking involved in the response to the outbreak is staggering and would be a serious test of global public health institutions even in the best of circumstances.

These are not the best of circumstances.

The international response to COVID-19 is happening amid one of the most precarious moments in diplomatic history. The United States has been escalating a trade war with China and applying geopolitical pressure through proxies. The United States was also on the brink of war with Iran just a few weeks ago. Now, all of these countries are experiencing significant increases in infections within their borders—and all three governments are facing significant criticism[12] for using the response to score political points instead of ending the outbreak.[13] The head of the World Health Organization (WHO) recently warned that the window to contain the epidemic is closing[14]—and some experts are suggesting it's time to prepare the public for a pandemic.[15]

113

Beyond specific geopolitical tensions, the news ecosystem surrounding the outbreak is unfolding amid historic concern over misinformation and disinformation. Already a number of states (and state-friendly platforms) are using the media to try to influence public opinion about the outbreak. Information was censored on Chinese social media platforms.[16] Russian state television spread the theory that Trump actually manufactured the disease.[17] And Rush Limbaugh, an American far-right commentator (and recent recipient of the Presidential Medal of Freedom), said that "this coronavirus thing" is a conspiracy to undermine Trump.[18] The trend of using global emergencies to make political points is hardly new, but because of the power of the internet, it's never been easier or more damaging. The WHO itself is facing challenges to its credibility for supporting China's response.[19]

Amidst rumours that Iran has lost control of the epidemic, Turkey and Pakistan have closed their borders.[20] The epidemic has surged in Italy and South Korea, leading both to implement large-scale quarantines over the weekend.[21] And the world economy is bracing for large negative impacts as spending, manufacturing, and travel all slow.[22] The US Stock Exchange reacted by having two of its worst days on record [during the last week of February 2020].[23]

The largest difference between an epidemic and a pandemic is the way we respond. Epidemic response focuses on isolation, surveillance and control—all in an effort to use social controls to contain and, hopefully, eliminate the pathogen. Pandemic response lets go of social controls, acknowledging their failure, and invests in public health infrastructure to begin systemic response. Large spikes in the number of infected in Italy, Iran, and South Korea are clear signs that we may be beyond containment.

It's worth asking ourselves, as information politics continues to define very real borders and markets, whether our approach to the infodemic is on a similar brink. The international policy community's focus on misinformation and disinformation, for the past several years, has focused on a strategy of containment and blame. As the consequences of disinformation during this emergency continue to escalate, so does the incentive to invest in the quality and governance of public information infrastructure. We may find that misinformation, much like this new virus, is beyond the world's powers to contain, and the best thing we can do is mobilize systems of digital diplomacy and adapt.

Unfortunately, the tools and tactics of social control that we develop during a public health crisis get repurposed, after the emergency, for political means. The social licence created to use call records, for example, has been repurposed for traffic analysis.[24] It's all too predictable that the digital tools, tactics and powers that we develop during this response will lead to future attempts to manipulate markets, borders and politics.

Often, great tragedy inspires reinvestments in shared standards and governance. Some of the most important international biomedical ethics laws and institutions were founded in the wake of World War II—based on the findings of the Nuremberg Doctors Trial and the resulting Belmont Report. While the effects of the COVID-19 outbreak can't be compared to the scale of mortality or global concern caused by World War II, it is worth asking what amount of disaster we'll need to endure in order to build public health information infrastructure that can be trusted.

This epidemic has come at a time when the world's diplomatic relations are strained. In this environment, strident digital, surveillance, and diplomatic policies are being written in the heat of a disaster—not through deliberation or agreement, but through escalating, unilateral declarations of protectionism. In addition to demonstrating the fragility of the world's public health and public information systems, the COVID-19 crisis is also exposing the fragility of international diplomacy and its digitalpolitik—the use of digital statecraft to advance political interests.[25] If the system is to heal, we'll have to invest in diplomacy—digital and otherwise—or the next disaster may do more than illustrate the system's fragility.

Notes

1 Karen Hao and Tanya Basu, "The Coronavirus Is the First True Social-Media 'Infodemic,'" *MIT Technology Review*, 12 February 2020.

2 "China Expels Three Wall Street Journal Reporters," *Wall Street Journal*, 19 February 2020.

3 Bethany Allen-Ebrahimian, "Exclusive: Pompeo Says New China Media Restrictions 'Long Overdue,'" *Axios*, 18 February 2020.

4 David McCabe, Nicole Hong, and Katie Benner, "US Charges Huawei with Racketeering, Adding Pressure on China," *New York Times*, 13 February 2020.

5 Nsikan Akpan, "Coronavirus Spikes outside China Show Travel Bans Aren't Working," *National Geographic*, 24 February 2020.

6 David Lim, "Problems with CDC Coronavirus Test Delay Expanded US Screening," *Politico*, 20 February 2020.

7 Jeyup S. Kwaak, "MERS: South Korea Tightens Quarantines to Prevent Spread," *Wall Street Journal*, 15 June 2015.

8 Sean Martin McDonald, "Ebola: A Big Data Disaster," *The Centre for Internet & Society*, 1 March 2016.

9 Jackie Salo, "Uber Suspends Hundreds of Accounts after Coronavirus Patient Takes Rides in Mexico," *New York Post*, 4 February 2020.

10 Michael Collins and John Fritze, "'No Need to Panic': President Trump Says Risk to Americans Is Low as First Coronavirus Death Reported in US," *USA Today*, 29 February 2020.

11 Ben Blanchard, "Taiwan Accuses China of Waging Cyber 'War' to Disrupt Virus Fight," *Reuters*, 29 February 2020.

12 Sam Jones, Aamna Mohdin, and agencies, "Coronavirus: Iran Denies Cover-Up as Six Deaths Reported in Italy," *Guardian*, 24 February 2020.

13 Alicia Cohn, "Trump Backs Off Plan to House Coronavirus Patients in Alabama after GOP Objections," *The Hill*, 24 February 2020.

14 "Coronavirus: 'Narrowing Window' to Contain Outbreak, WHO Says," *BBC News*, 22 February 2020.

15 Julia Belluz, "'We Are at a Turning Point': The Coronavirus Outbreak Is Looking More like a Pandemic," *Vox*, 25 February 2020.

16 Li Yuan, "China Silences Critics over Deadly Virus Outbreak," *New York Times*, 22 January 2020.

17 "Russian TV Runs Conspiracy Theory Blaming Trump for Coronavirus," *Moscow Times*, 7 February 2020.

18 "Overhyped Coronavirus Weaponized against Trump," *Rush Limbaugh Show*, 24 February 2020.

19 Emily Rauhala, "Chinese Officials Note Serious Problems in Coronavirus Response. The World Health Organization Keeps Praising Them," *Washington Post*, 8 February 2020.

20 Patrick Wintour, "Turkey and Pakistan Close Borders with Iran over Coronavirus Deaths," *Guardian*, 23 February 2020.

21 "Coronavirus: South Korea Declares Highest Alert as Infections Surge," *BBC News*, 23 February 2020.

22 Rosamond Hutt, "The Economic Effects of COVID-19 around the World," *World Economic Forum*, 17 February 2020.

23 William Watts and Sunny Oh, "Dow Bounces Nearly 1,300 Points as Stocks End Sharply Higher following Worst Week since 2008," *MarketWatch*, 2 March 2020.

24 "Mobile Big Data Solutions for a Better Future," *GSMA*, 2019.

25 Sean McDonald and An Xiao Mina, "The War-Torn Web," *Foreign Policy*, 19 December 2018.

CASE STUDY

Physician-Patient Privilege vs. Public Health Policy

Dr. Mary Samson is a family practitioner in a small and neighborly New England town. She has been the family doctor of Karl and Ayat, a couple in their mid-thirties, for 10 years. Three months ago, COVID-19 emerged and spread rapidly through the country, but as yet no cases have surfaced in the quiet, close-knit town.

Karl owns an auto parts supply store and spends a couple of days each week delivering parts to mechanics in the region. A week ago, though, without telling Ayat, he called in sick and drove to New York. He spent the day there with Kate, an old girlfriend he'd reconnected with online, and within a week of his return he'd developed a slight fever, a nagging cough, and unusual chest pains.

He called Dr. Samson and she in turn asked both him and Ayat, who was asymptomatic, to come in for an appointment. During Karl's appointment, the weight of his recklessness overwhelmed him and he told Dr. Samson that he'd had an affair. He implored her not to say anything to Ayat and made a direct appeal to patient-physician confidentiality. Indeed, Karl told Dr. Samson that he wouldn't have said anything about his affair if he hadn't believed that this information was protected by requirements of confidentiality.

Dr. Samson referred Karl and Ayat for COVID-19 testing straight away, and both tests came back positive. Soon thereafter, the regional public health authority scheduled interviews to begin contact tracing—the process of identifying people who've been in contact with the infected. When Karl learned of the interview, he called Dr. Samson, frantic with worry. By sheer coincidence, Brenda, a close friend of Karl and Ayat's, had recently volunteered to help with contact tracing.

Karl told Dr. Samson that he planned not to reveal his New York trip or his contact with Kate to the contact tracing authorities because he feared that this information would in one way or another reach Brenda and then potentially leak out to Ayat and other friends, family, and coworkers. He assured Dr. Samson that he'd told Kate of his diagnosis and that she had arranged for testing and was self-isolating. He also said that he'd interacted with no one else during his New York trip and so he wouldn't be hiding any other contact information from the authorities

Dr. Samson was faced with a decision. Should she caution the authorities that Karl might withhold information in his interview? If she did so, Karl could face the prospect of serious criminal charges. She felt that Brenda probably wouldn't discover the affair if the authorities were notified, but she wasn't sure, as she knew little about the technical details of contact tracing. She knew as well that some recent health-care policies seemed to waive or diminish certain ordinary requirements of patient confidentiality.[1] The chances of Ayat finding out were probably low but certainly not infinitesimal, especially if Karl were to face reprimand for lying to the health authorities.

Dr. Samson took her "duty to warn"[2] extremely seriously. But she also felt keenly her obligation to protect Karl's confidentiality. She found his behavior repugnant; but she was his doctor, after all, not his judge. Additionally, she was concerned that data collection was itself fraught. The very possibility that Brenda could stumble upon details demonstrated the complications inherent in promised anonymity. Not to mention: Could anyone guarantee how the information might be used in the future? Weren't security breaches possible?

Karl was obviously under the impression that the principle of confidentiality was inviolable. He would have said nothing to Dr. Samson if he suspected otherwise. Dr. Samson worried that if she and other health-care workers disregarded this expectation of confidentiality it could have a "chilling" effect, in that patients would then be less forthcoming with important information. Should this enter into Dr. Samson's decision?

Karl argued that the outcome was the same whether or not he told the authorities, because he'd separately informed Kate of his diagnosis. Should Dr. Samson consider this argument, or is she obligated to abide by the rules regardless of her belief about the likely outcome?

Do standard requirements of patient confidentiality weaken in the face of a pandemic or other health-care crisis?

Notes

1   The Health Insurance Portability and Accountability Act (HIPAA) of 1996 established procedures for maintaining the privacy of individuals' health information and instituted civil and criminal penalties for violations. In March 2020, the United States Department of Health and Human Services released a bulletin in response to COVID-19 that waived these HIPAA penalties during nationwide public health emergencies. Public health authorities and health-care providers were therefore permitted to disclose protected health information without individual authorization, provided they "make reasonable efforts to limit the information disclosed to that which is the 'minimum necessary' to accomplish the purpose."

2   Standards for a "duty to warn" (or "duty to protect") in the United States were established with the *Tarasoff* case in 1976. Initially, it pertained to psychiatrists' duty to warn about clients' potentially violent behavior, but it gradually expanded (especially during the HIV outbreak) to cover physical medicine as well. Guidelines for reporting vary considerably by state, ranging from statutorily mandated laws to no statutory guidance whatsoever. Many states' guidelines include determining whether or not the harm prevented by the breach of confidentiality would outweigh the harm caused by the breach of confidentiality.

QUESTIONS FOR REFLECTION

1. Are there ways to introduce programs that involve massive surveillance at a national and global level while still protecting privacy and liberty? Could the careful and restricted introduction of these programs enhance our privacy and liberty in the long run, as Cegłowski suggests?

2. Thompson and Cegłowski frame the moral dilemma involved in limiting privacy differently. Identify the moral dilemma as framed by each of them. How does the different framing affect their evaluations of the limits to privacy?

3. In ordinary circumstances outside of a pandemic, do individual citizens have a right to privacy when it comes to matters of public health? Would it be morally acceptable for a government to track suspected infections of non-pandemic diseases such as influenza or herpes using GPS surveillance and other such techniques, if doing so proved to be effective in reducing the incidence of those diseases?

4. Does it make a moral difference whether the adoption of a surveillance program is voluntary or mandatory? If a government were to strongly encourage the use of a surveillance app but not require it, would this count as an infringement on privacy at all?

5. Do individuals have a moral obligation to download and use contact tracing apps? Would you voluntarily use a contact tracing app? Would you strongly encourage your friends and family members to do the same? What moral values guide your decision?

8

Reopening

INTRODUCTION

Before the COVID-19 pandemic began, I would joke about how I wished I could stay home and do nothing for an extended period of time. One of the things that's surprised me the most about this pandemic is just how difficult it is do nothing. Humans are social creatures, and staying away from others can cause anxiety, depression, loneliness and other mental, physical, and emotional challenges. After only a few weeks of physical distancing, many people began to long for a reopening of society—visiting friends and family, going to work, and engaging in other daily social activities.

Quite apart from that, there are also powerful economic reasons to reopen, and these aren't just abstract concerns about GDP or stock value. There are immediate and pressing worries from countless small-business owners whose livelihoods are threatened by prolonged shutdown, and from financially vulnerable people who need either financial aid or a return to work in order to pay their rent and grocery bills. Prolonged shutdowns in wealthy parts of the world can also have disastrous effects on poorer nations, whose industries depend on sales to wealthy countries.

Yet it seems that it is easier to close things down than it is to reopen them. Evidence from countries around the world suggests that reopening, even when done carefully, can cause an increase of infection. And we know from historical examples, including the 1918–19 flu pandemic, that the second wave can be more deadly than the first. Nevertheless, this virus is novel and has proven to be difficult to predict. This is the first known coronavirus pandemic, so our history with other pandemics might prove an unreliable guide.

This chapter opens with a reading by Arthur Caplan, who argues that it is immoral to talk about reopening the economy before the pandemic is under control, as saving lives is more important than wealth maximization. Caplan recognizes that economic downturns also have negative effects on health and mortality, but he claims that we do not yet know enough about SARS-CoV-2 to reopen safely. He holds that slow economic recovery is not worth the cost in human lives.

Conor Friedersdorf highlights the difficulty of making choices about whether to reopen or stay closed, as both options involve considerable harms under conditions of extreme uncertainty. Friedersdorf notes that the debate around whether to loosen self-isolation measures is often framed in terms of saving human lives or saving the economy. He suggests that the issues are not so straightforward, as economic shutdowns also have negative effects on our survival and well-being. The health effects of COVID-19 are felt immediately, but the effects of economic shutdowns might be with us for years to come.

In the third reading of this chapter, Daniel Weinstock offers a creative harm reduction approach to reopening. Since it is not possible to continue current practices of physical distancing and social isolation indefinitely, it may be necessary to find practical ways of loosening regulations while reducing interpersonal contact. Weinstock suggests that we rethink our use of time and space. The early response to the pandemic tended to constrict both time and space by closing public areas and restricting the hours of grocery stores and parks. Weinstock suggests we could better achieve the goals of physical distancing by taking the opposite approach: opening as many spaces to the public as possible, and allowing people to work and socialize throughout the whole 24 hours of the day. This would allow us to better spread ourselves out over time and space, thereby maintaining our distance.

Tied in with the issue of reopening is the hope that we may create a vaccine for COVID-19 in the near future. If an effective vaccine is developed, however, there will remain questions of implementation: how should it be applied to the public, and should it be mandatory? In the final reading of this book, Anthony Skelton and Lisa Forsberg provide several arguments in support of mandatory vaccination protocols.

As of late May 2020, many of the suggestions found in this chapter are untested. We are not yet sure how we will get out of the current pandemic slowdown or how successful our attempts at reopening will be. The readings give a glimpse of our thinking while we are still in the midst of stay-at-home recommendations.

KEY TERMS

harm reduction: a type of public health policy that attempts to reduce the harms caused by a given behavior or problem while acknowledging that the behavior is not likely to be eliminated. Common examples of harm reduction are the creation of "safe injection" sites for users of heroin and other drugs (as opposed to the criminalization of drug possession) and the provision of sexual health advice and prophylactics in schools (as opposed to the insistence on abstinence).

herd immunity: a state in which a population has heightened resistance to an infectious disease. Herd immunity occurs when a substantial number of members within a given population are immune to a disease, typically because they've either been vaccinated or developed antibodies as a result of prior exposure. Once a population achieves herd immunity, an infectious disease will be unlikely to spread within that population because the individuals susceptible to infection will be few and far between.

8.1

The Price of Going Back to Work Too Soon

Arthur Caplan

President Donald Trump had, until very recently [6 April 2020], spent as much time in his public appearances proclaiming victory over the COVID-19 pandemic rippling across the nation as he had offering directives that would diminish it. Again and again, he promised that it would soon be over, especially as the weather got warmer, and that the worst would not happen or was already behind us. This triggered a widespread discussion that still is ongoing about how fast America could get back to normal and get the economy roaring again.

But even floating the notion of reopening the economy was grossly immoral. Why?

I take outcomes very seriously. Morally trying to do what is best for the greatest number is what guides my thinking about how to allocate ventilators or reopen the economy. But for me, wealth maximization is not as important a goal as saving huge numbers of lives. And talk of back to normal to salvage the economy before the pandemic is stabilized does not add up.

It is true that Trump is not alone in plumping for the economy. A lot of serious people are concerned about the downstream effects of the economic shutdown. Many leaders around the world worry about how disrupted supply chains could lead to longer-term poverty, social turmoil and disease. Talk has resumed in China, Italy, South Korea, and the city of Hong Kong about releasing people from isolation.

The problem is there are still too many unknowns to predict the numbers of when it is time to put the economy ahead of the risk of further deaths. We don't know if those who have been infected can be reinfected. We don't know if the virus can incubate in a locality and then roar back. We don't know what level of antibodies means you might be protected but still could infect others since we really don't know what the safe incubation period is. And we still don't have enough tests so that we can do the kind of constant checking and isolating of the positive that would let the desire to get back to business occur. Worse, many parts of the world are still isolating or yet to be infected, meaning at best a slow partial economic return is in store.

Those who dismiss the potential for mass casualities, nonexistent health care systems and huge numbers of dead police, firemen, truck drivers, and day care workers as opposed to putting the economy on hold for three more months are engaged in morally perverse mathematics. The price of going back to work too soon or reigniting the plague is not balanced by gradual and slow economic activity.

And there is a different damage caused by irresponsible talk of "back to business" in days, weeks, by Easter or by Memorial Day. Such debate strongly undermines the resolve that Americans need to adhere to recommendations to stay at home as much as possible and maintain physical distance from others. If things will soon be better, then how bad can a trip to visit grandma, heading down to the beach in big groups, inviting kids over for playdates or going camping with 400 other people be? Many Americans are not isolating, and talk of starting up soon is not likely to motivate them to do so.

Rather than rebuild an economy on hiatus around the world for months, we will find ourselves trying to spark a wounded economy for years if we don't answer the key viral infectivity questions first. A rich nation can work through an economic shutdown of months. A broken and devastated nation beset by new outbreaks and constant conflicting messages about the need for isolation will not regain a sound economy for years, if ever.

8.2

Take the Shutdown Skeptics Seriously

Conor Friedersdorf

Should states ease pandemic restrictions or extend lockdowns and shelter-in-place orders into the summer? That question confronts leaders across the United States. President Trump says that "we have to get our country open." And many governors are moving quickly in that direction.

Critics are dismayed. Citing forecasts that COVID-19 deaths could rise to 3,000 per day in June, they say that reopening without better defenses against infections is reckless. That assessment may well be correct. Many insist it is immoral, too. The columnist Amy Z. Quinn says the Trump administration is "choosing money over lives."[1] In a CNN news analysis, Daniel Burke offers this characterization of America's choice: "Should we reopen the economy to help the majority or protect the lives of the vulnerable?"

Denunciations of that sort cast the lockdown debate as a straightforward battle between a pro-human and a pro-economy camp. But the actual trade-offs are not straightforward. Set aside "flattening the curve," which will continue to make sense. Are ongoing, onerous shutdowns warranted *beyond* what is necessary to avoid overwhelming ambulances, hospitals, and morgues?

The answer depends in part on an unknown: how close the country is to containing the virus.

"The public, the media, the business community, and policymakers are largely unprepared for a pessimistic scenario," the Foundation for Research on Equal Opportunity argued in a recent white paper. That is, the US may have no treatment, no vaccine, and no ability to scale up testing and quarantining, due to technical hurdles or Trump administration incompetence or a lack of public buy-in.

If we knew that a broadly effective COVID-19 treatment was imminent, or that a working vaccine was months away, minimizing infections through social distancing until that moment would be the right course. At the other extreme, if we will never have an effective treatment or vaccine and most everyone will get infected eventually, then the costs of social distancing are untenable. We don't *know* where we sit on that spectrum. So we cannot *know* what the best way forward is even if we place the highest possible value on preserving life and protecting the vulnerable.

125

That uncertainty means, at the very least, that Americans should carefully consider the potential costs of prolonged shutdowns lest they cause more deaths or harm to the vulnerable than they spare.

Ongoing closures and supply-chain interruptions in wealthier countries could have catastrophic ripple effects, Michael T. Klare warns in *The Nation*, highlighting the possibility that global starvation could soar. "Even where supply chains remain intact, many poor countries lack the funds to pay for imported food," he explained.[2] "This has long been a problem for the least-developed countries, which often depend on international food aid...It is becoming even more severe as the number of people without jobs multiplies and donor countries balk at higher aid expenditures." His article wasn't a brief for reopening the economy, but it implied a need to guard against shutdowns that cause more deaths via starvation than are saved by slowing infections.

"A prolonged depression will stunt lives as surely as any viral epidemic, and its toll will not be confined to the elderly," Heather Mac Donald argues at *Spectator USA*.[3] "The shuttering of auto manufacturing plants led to an 85 percent increase in opioid overdose deaths in the surrounding counties over seven years, according to a recent study." Deficit spending may be necessary to keep people afloat, she continued, but the wealth that permits it could quickly evaporate. "The enormously complex web of trade, once killed, cannot be brought back to life by government stimulus. And who is going to pay for all that deficit spending as businesses close and tax revenues disappear?"

At *Arc Digital*, Esther O'Reilly asks, "Why should we assume that a crashing economy would leave the healthcare system standing?"[4] Fleshing out the matter, she writes, "You can't keep the hospital lights on without keeping on the lights of the economic sectors undergirding it. Yes, our doctors and nurses are running out of masks and gloves, which is a serious problem. It would also be a serious problem if we lost the means and the manpower to make more, or if the hospitals ran out of cash on hand to buy more beds, ventilators, etc. And there's the rub. We are being told we can't fight the virus without pausing the economy, yet we can't fight the virus without the economy."

School closures may do long-term damage, as well. A recent study in *The Lancet* concluded that "the evidence for the effectiveness of school closures and other school social distancing measures comes almost entirely from influenza outbreaks," and that the effectiveness of school measures in a coronavirus outbreak is uncertain.[5] [The study also] noted that "education is one of the strongest predictors of the health and the wealth of a country's future workers, and the impact of long-term school closure on educational outcomes, future earnings, the health of young people, and future national productivity has not been quantified." A given closure could add months to the lives of some *and* subtract from the lives of others.

The general point is that minimizing the number of COVID-19 deaths today or a month from now or six months from now may *or may not* minimize the human costs of the pandemic when the full spectrum of human consequences is considered. The last global depression created conditions for a catastrophic world war that killed roughly 75 to 80 million people. Is that a possibility? The downside risks and costs of every approach are real, frightening, and depressing, no matter how little one thinks of reopening now.

These facts may not be evident from the least thoughtful proponents of re-opening, many of whom advance arguments that are uninformed, dismissive of experts, or callous. But the warnings of *thoughtful* shutdown skeptics warrant careful study, not stigma rooted in the false pretense that they don't have any plausible concerns or value human life.

Notes

1 Amy Z. Quinn, "Trump Is Choosing Sides in Coronavirus Battle: Money over Lives," *NJ.com*, 30 April 2020.
2 Michael T. Klare, "COVID-19's Third Shock Wave: The Global Food Crisis," *The Nation*, 1 May 2020.
3 Heather Mac Donald, "Consider the Costs," *Spectator USA*, 22 March 2020.
4 Esther O'Reilly, "Economic Costs Are Human Costs," *Arc Digital*, 25 March 2020.
5 Russell M. Viner, et al., "School Closure and Management Practices during Coronavirus Outbreaks Including COVID-19: A Rapid Systematic Review," *The Lancet: Child & Adolescent Health*, vol. 4, no. 5, 1 May 2020.

8.3

A Harm Reduction Approach to Physical Distancing

Daniel Weinstock

The Physical Distancing Dilemma

If, like me, you spend an inordinate amount of time poring over the research that is being generated in record time in the context of the COVID-19 pandemic by researchers in a wide array of disciplines, you will know that uncertainties abound. What's more, they abound across a wide range of dimensions. Models predicting rates of infection are propounded and quickly discarded, estimations of the likelihood of a vaccine range from the optimistic to the cautionary.

In such a context, we need to make plans that cover a wide range of fact patterns. I want to begin thinking about one such pattern. What if it turns out that we need to engage in physical distancing for the next couple of years, or maybe even indefinitely? Unless there are significant advances in the treatment of COVID-19, distancing is likely to be required until a vaccine is discovered, manufactured at a planetary scale, and administered at a sufficient scale to ensure some degree of collective immunity. And if we don't discover a vaccine, we'll probably have to engage in distancing for longer. Keeping the curve flat enough so as not to overwhelm our health systems until we achieve herd immunity could take years. And if having gone through COVID-19 does not confer immunity, then....

If physical distancing requires that the kind of confinement we have been undergoing for the past few weeks extends into the indefinite future, it is going to be a tough sell. As warm weather returns to Canada, the risk is that Canadians will "vote with their feet," and observe stay at home orders in an increasingly lax way. As they do, the ability of law enforcement to effectively enforce a stay at home policy will quickly be overtaxed. Should we then just give up on physical distancing? Do we end up defaulting to the reviled model according to which we just throw up our hands and let the virus make its way through our communities, resulting in staggering numbers of deaths?

A Harm Reduction Approach

Not necessarily. The kind of scenario that I have just mooted is structurally familiar to those of us who are interested in "harm reduction" models. The circumstances of harm reduction are ones in which we come to realize that it is impossible to enforce the prohibition of some mode of behaviour that is either controversial or outright condemnable, or at least not possible at acceptable cost. Partisans of harm reduction approaches claim that the continued attempt to enforce prohibitions lead to the worst of all possible worlds, a kind of unregulated non-compliance, if you will.

Sufficient compliance with stay-at-home policies will be very difficult to maintain and to enforce, and it will get increasingly difficult as lockdowns extend, from weeks, to months, to possibly years. If physical distancing is equated with staying at home unless it is absolutely necessary to leave, then we are in trouble.

Moreover, the concerns that physical isolation policies raise are not just about the growing gulf between our willingness to comply and the ability to enforce. There are moral costs as well. "Stay at home" is a massively inegalitarian response to the pandemic, because it distributes the burdens of combatting the virus so unequally. Some people get to stay home while still being paid, in nice houses with family members and partners with whom they get along. Others live in cramped spaces, or cohabit with abusive partners, and/or end up losing their livelihoods and so have to make do in increasingly straitened economic circumstances. It's one thing to accept this inegalitarian policy as a short, sharp shock, to get us over the first wave of the pandemic. It is quite another to require it over the long haul. It involves putting the mental and physical health of some of our most vulnerable citizens at risk.

So we seem to have hit an impasse. In the absence of a pharmaceutical or technological fix, the most plausible policy response we have is both impracticable and unacceptably inegalitarian over the long haul.

Stretching Space

But there may be a way out. One possibility whose full potential has perhaps not yet been fully explored is that physical distancing does not require confinement, or at least not as much confinement as has been required thus far. This possibility would involve making a much more efficient use of time and of space in our organization of work and leisure, so that we can, as it were, spread people out as they go about their activities in a way that respects social distancing requirements.

Think, first, of space. A reaction of many municipal governments in the face of COVID-19 has been to close off green spaces, or to render them inaccessible. For example, in Montreal, the parking lots of Mount-Royal park have been closed, which makes the park for all intents and purposes inaccessible to a vast proportion of Montrealers. Similar policies have been enacted in other jurisdictions, where vast expanses such as parking lots and schoolyards have been closed off.

Presumably, the thinking is that if you close these spaces off, you make going out less attractive to people, and they will then be more inclined to comply with "stay at home" restrictions. But the other possibility, one that risks becoming more likely as time goes by, is that people will go out, but that they will do so in spaces such as narrow sidewalks in which they are far less likely to be able to comply with physical distancing requirements than they would be in wide, open spaces.

In Montreal, this risk has already been tacitly recognized by city officials, who have widened the area in which people are able to walk by eliminating at least one side of streets' parking spaces. There's a tension here: on the one hand, officials want to make attractive spaces inaccessible to disincentivize people going out, but on the other they recognize that they will go out, and so they make the spaces that are left to them more compatible with distancing requirements.

The harm reduction thinking that is implicit in the latter set of measures should in my view be fully embraced. We should make spaces more widely available, rather than less, so that people can spread themselves out in ways that make physical distancing possible.

We should consider doing this not just with outdoor, but with indoor spaces as well. Those of our fellow citizens who do not have access to safe, adequate housing should be able to access currently unused spaces (theatres, cinemas, hotels) where distancing requirements could be enforced, in order to work, to study, or simply to take a break from unsafe home conditions.

The basic idea is: if you need to space people out, use as much of the space that there is!

Rethinking Time

Researchers in Australia have argued in a recent piece that we should think about time in the same way, and I agree. Our society has evolved so that almost everyone has largely convergent work and leisure schedules. Everyone works, roughly, from 9 to 5. Every child goes to school, roughly, from 8 to 3 or thereabouts. As anyone who has ever driven a car or taken public transport to work, or tried to get lunch in a downtown food court knows, this creates temporal jams. There are times in the day where temporal convergence forces us into densely packed crowds. In recent decades we have started experimenting with flexible work schedules, but this is still a marginal phenomenon.

Just as we don't use space as efficiently as we might in order to achieve physical distancing, so we don't use the 24-hour clock or the 7-day week as efficiently as we might to achieve the same end. We are already toying with the thought that deconfinement will require creative uses of time. For example, it has been suggested here in Quebec that when schools reopen, the school day will be organized in such a way that children will never all be at school at the same time. There will be a morning and an afternoon shift. The plausible thought is that if you spread out the day and distribute kids across it, rather than lumping them all in the same 6–7 hour slot, you make distancing more possible.

At the same time, jurisdictions have had the opposite temporal reflex. Curfews have been imposed, and in Quebec, Sunday has been re-imposed as a day of rest even for certain essential services, such as grocery stores. While the impetus behind this is intelligible, it makes little sense if our goal is to maximize opportunities for physical distancing. Spread the same number of people out over longer periods of time, and the chance that they will be able to distance without having to confine grows. Rather than restricting the times during which people can access the spaces that they need to be in, why not extend them? For the length of the pandemic, keep stores, workplaces, and yes, perhaps even schools open 24/7, and distribute people in sparser, and more distancing-enabling ways.

Get Out of the Box

Unimaginable? Perhaps. But the present set of circumstances, and the responses that we have enacted to them, would have seemed unimaginable just a few short weeks ago. The predicament we find ourselves in requires out-of-the box think-ing, especially under the moderately pessimistic conditions that I have identified as premises for this intervention.

Obviously, we will need planners and architects to help us figure out the de-tails of how to re-organize our institutions, our spaces and our communities. But the basic point stands. If we want to achieve long-term physical distancing, "stay at home" cannot be the solution. It exacerbates inequality, and in any case is probably only achievable given a massive uptake in surveillance and coercion by the state, and snitching on the part of ordinary citizens, which would leave an unattractive stain on our post-pandemic lives.

8.4

Mandating Vaccination

Anthony Skelton and Lisa Forsberg

The race to develop a vaccine for COVID-19 is on. Finding a vaccine is the most promising route to lifting the public health restrictions currently in place to pre-vent the spread of coronavirus, which has already killed hundreds of thousands of people and infected many more. It is possible that a viable vaccine candidate may emerge in the not-too-distant future.

At the height of the pandemic, Canadian prime minister Justin Trudeau was asked whether he would mandate vaccination for COVID-19. He replied that "we still have a fair bit of time to reflect on … [the best vaccination protocol] in order to get it right." But the time to reflect is now. The legislative changes needed to develop and implement a policy are complex. Reflecting on the policy options and their moral justification will put us in the best position to select the most ef-fective one available. Here we reflect on some arguments for a mandatory scheme (for other arguments, see Brennan, 2018; Flanigan, 2014; Giubilini, forthcoming; and Giubilini et al., 2018).

There is some enthusiasm in several jurisdictions (including in Italy, Canada, and the United States) for mandating that parents vaccinate their children. In these jurisdictions, parents are (with some exceptions) required to vaccinate their (young) children in order for them to attend school or daycare.

Might the best arguments in favor of mandating the vaccination of children also lend support to mandating vaccination more generally?

One of the most compelling arguments for mandating the vaccination of children rests on the claim that sending unvaccinated children to school involves imposing a very significant risk of death and suffering on other children, especially those who cannot be vaccinated for medical reasons. The argument runs as follows. If, by vaccinating their children, parents can easily and safely avoid imposing a significant risk of death and suffering on other children, parents ought to vaccinate their children. Vaccinating one's children is an easy and safe way to avoid imposing the risk of death and suffering on other children; vaccination poses only a very small risk to those who are vaccinated. The state has an obligation to protect children from exposure to easily avoidable risk of death and suffering. Therefore, the state ought to mandate that parents vaccinate their children.

The same reasoning might justify a mandatory vaccination scheme for adults. Anyone who is not vaccinated poses a risk to others, especially to the most vulnerable. Individuals can easily and without much cost to themselves avoid posing a significant risk to others. If assuming a small cost in order to avoid posing a great risk to others is sufficient to justify preventing parents from taking advantage of school and daycare, would it not also be sufficient to justify mandatory vaccination more generally?

A second argument in favor of mandating the vaccination of children goes as follows. Parents or guardians are not permitted to expose their children to substantial risk of death and suffering when it is easy to avoid doing so. Parents who do not vaccinate their children against serious illnesses expose their children to such risks. It is impermissible, then, for parents not to vaccinate their children against serious illness (unless there are medical reasons against vaccination). The state has an obligation to protect children from exposure to easily avoidable risk of death and suffering. Therefore, the state ought to mandate the vaccination of children (Pierik, 2018). If the COVID-19 vaccine is as safe and effective as, say, the measles vaccine, then there is a low-risk way to avoid an infection that may cause death or serious suffering. The state ought to mandate that parents vaccinate their children against COVID-19.

This is a compelling argument for mandatory vaccination of children, but it may not easily translate to the case of adults, because it is generally accepted that there are important differences between children and adults that justify differences in treatment of each class. Children, at least when young, are not autonomous and do not have decision-making capacity. When an individual is not autonomous or does not have decision-making capacity, it is generally taken to be permissible to treat her in her best interests. If a vaccine is safe and effective in preventing an infectious disease that carries significant risks of death or serious suffering, there seems to be compelling reason to vaccinate individuals lacking decision-making capacity on grounds of their best interests—whether the individuals in question are children or adults.

But when adults possess decision-making capacity, it is generally taken to be impermissible to treat them paternalistically. Such adults are generally taken to have a robust right to refuse medical interventions even when those interventions are clearly in their best interests and when not undergoing the interventions will lead to their death or serious suffering. While the vaccination of children might be justified on grounds of their best interests, vaccination of adults who possess decision-making capacity would be hard to justify *on grounds of their best interests* on many moral views.

There is perhaps one way in which the second argument might, in a fashion similar to the first argument above, generate a case in favor of mandating vaccination for all. The reason the state has for preventing parents from inflicting risk of death or serious illness on their children might be that the state has a more general duty to protect the vulnerable. If this is the reason for mandating the vaccination of children, it might provide justification for a general scheme for mandatory vaccination. A mandatory vaccination scheme for everyone protects very young children and those unable to be vaccinated for medical reasons. If the protection of the vulnerable is a reason to mandate the vaccination of children, why is it not also a reason to mandate vaccination more generally (at least for serious conditions like COVID-19)?

A third argument for mandating the vaccination of children turns on differences between adults and children in terms of the nature of their well-being. Children might fare well in a different way than adults (Skelton, 2018; Wendler, 2012). It is plausible that what matters most to the well-being of adults is their subjective attitudes (authentic happiness or the satisfaction of their rational desires). This may not be true of (especially young) children. While happiness and the satisfaction of desires matters to children's well-being, it might not be what matters most. Perhaps so-called "objective goods" (things that make one better off without satisfying a desire or making one happier) play a significant role in children's well-being, for example, valuable relationships and intellectual engagement.

Suppose that one such objective good lies in making a contribution in some way to some socially worthwhile endeavor (like research with the potential to find a cure for a serious disease). A child might do this by being enrolled as a research subject (Wendler, 2012). Making a causal contribution to societal herd immunity that protects the vulnerable might be one such good. If being vaccinated causally contributes to the good of herd immunity and protection of the vulnerable, it might be good for children to be vaccinated.

This might justify mandating the vaccination of children but not adults, on the assumption that what is good for adults is determined by their subjective attitudes alone. For adults who find no happiness or desire satisfaction in being part of socially valuable practices, it might not be good for them to participate in socially worthwhile endeavors like the creation of herd immunity. But many adults do, and more might revise their subjective attitudes to desire or take happiness in being vaccinated when properly informed of how socially worthwhile the creation of herd immunity is. And, of course, if it turns out that the well-being of adults is enhanced by objective goods, including the good of contributing to socially worthwhile endeavors or something similar, it will be good for adults *and* children to be vaccinated.

It may be that making vaccination mandatory would increase resistance to it, either by making more people unwilling to undergo vaccination or by making some people more determined not to undergo it. This, some have suggested, could lead to lower vaccination rates under a scheme that mandates vaccination than under one in which vaccination is voluntary.

If, empirically speaking, instituting a mandatory vaccination scheme led to a reduction in vaccination rates, we might have to concede that a scheme of this sort would not be, all things considered, best. If mandatory vaccination schemes face resistance, it may be better to use nudges or some other mechanism to encourage individuals to vaccinate themselves and their children. It is worth noting, though, that this type of "resistance effect"—if real—might apply to alternatives to vaccination, such as lockdown or physical distancing measures, too, if these involved some element of coercion. It is not obvious, then, that a mandatory vaccination scheme would fare worse on this score than other coercive measures. Governments should therefore at least consider making vaccination mandatory, based on a comparison of the costs and benefits of the full range of available pandemic control measures.

References

Brennan, Jason (2018). "A Libertarian Case for Mandatory Vaccination." *Journal of Medical Ethics* 44, pp. 37–43.

Flanigan, Jessica (2014). "A Defense of Compulsory Vaccination." *HEC Forum* 26, pp. 5–25.

Giubilini, Alberto (forthcoming). "An Argument for Compulsory Vaccination: The Taxation Analogy." *Journal of Applied Philosophy.* https://doi.org/10.1111/japp.12400.

Giubilini, Alberto, et al. (2018). "The Moral Obligation to Be Vaccinated: Utilitarianism, Contractualism, and Collective Easy Rescue." *Medicine, Health Care, and Philosophy* 21, pp. 547–60.

Pierik, Roland (2018). "Mandatory Vaccination: An Unqualified Defence." *Journal of Applied Philosophy* 35, pp. 381–98.

Skelton, Anthony (2018). "Children and Well-being." In Anca Gheaus, Gideon Calder, & Jurgen De Wispelaere (eds.), *The Routledge Handbook of the Philosophy of Childhood and Children* (pp. 90–100). London: Routledge.

Wendler, David (2012). "A New Justification for Pediatric Research without the Potential for Clinical Benefit." *American Journal of Bioethics* 12, pp. 23–31.

CASE STUDY

Choosing Not to Vaccinate

Marlene Ford and her husband Brice have three children, aged six to ten. The Fords are relatively well off, and their children attend an exclusive private school called Hampton Hall. Marlene has kept to her children's vaccine schedules, even though she has some concerns about the involvement of large pharmaceutical companies in the vaccine industry. She realizes that vaccines are an important and life-saving medical tool. In general, Marlene follows the advice of doctors and other health-care authorities, both for herself and for her children. She also tries to protect her children's health through other means, such as by exposing them to dirt with the goal of building their immune capacity and by feeding them healthy foods.

Marlene has tried to abide faithfully to the physical distancing measures that have been put in place in her state as a response to the COVID-19 pandemic. She believes that public health doctors know what they are talking about when they give recommendations. She has sewn masks for herself, her family, and her friends, and she's donated additional masks to charities and the local hospital.

A vaccine for SARS-CoV-2 has now been developed, and public health officials are recommending that all children and adults be inoculated before they return to normal activities. Once inoculated, people will receive documents called "immunization records," which prove that they have been vaccinated and are safe to return to unrestricted movement. The vaccine is not mandated, and individuals are free to refuse vaccination for themselves or their children; however, if an individual refuses to be vaccinated for a non-medical reason, they will not be granted an immunization record and will not be permitted to leave social isolation. Unvaccinated children are not allowed to visit their friends, go to parks, or return to school. Unvaccinated adults are not able to return to workplaces or socialize with friends or family.

Marlene is eager to return to the activities of daily life, and she agrees that vaccination will most likely protect her children. However, she is concerned about the speed with which the SARS-CoV-2 vaccine was developed. The vaccine trials skipped several standard stages (such as animal studies) and were fast-tracked in human populations. Marlene is not sure that sufficient research has been conducted; she is concerned that, unlike other vaccines that have been in use for many years, this vaccine has not been adequately tested for long-term side-effects. She also knows that politicians and business leaders have encouraged the vaccine's fast-tracked development, and she worries that economic interests may have trumped considerations of public health in the vaccine's rapid testing and deployment.

Marlene's friend Rebecca has long been opposed to vaccines—not just the SARS-CoV-2 vaccine but also standard vaccinations for diseases such as measles, hepatitis-B, and influenza. Rebecca believes that the materials used to make vaccines are toxic and that they can cause autism and other health conditions. Because of this, she has not vaccinated her own children. Marlene knows that Rebecca's beliefs aren't grounded in good science and that they endanger her own family and others. Rebecca tells Marlene that she knows someone who works in public health and is involved in manufacturing the immunization record. Rebecca says that she can get forged immunization record for Marlene's entire family, which would allow them to live their lives unrestricted without getting vaccinated. Rebecca herself has already taken advantage of this, and she shows Marlene her forged immunization record, which looks entirely convincing.

Marlene disagrees with Rebecca's reasoning about vaccination in general, but she is nonetheless concerned about this particular vaccine due to its accelerated development. She also suspects that her family would be safe without vaccination, because if nearly everyone else receives the vaccine then the population will have herd immunity and the disease will cease to spread. Marlene believes that taking Rebecca up on her offer might lead to the best possible outcome for her family: they wouldn't likely become infected so long as herd immunity is established, and they wouldn't risk any possibility of long-term side-effects resulting from the vaccine. Assuming the vaccine proves to be safe in the long run, they can simply get vaccinated at a later point.

What should Marlene do? Should she accept the offer of forged documents if she believes that this is the safest path for her family? Keep in mind that Marlene's reasoning depends on the assumption that nearly everyone else *will* be vaccinated. If, on the other hand, each person makes themselves an exception, it's certain that the population will not obtain herd immunity and they will all be at serious risk.

Marlene has followed the news stories regarding COVID-19 and the development of the vaccine, but she also realizes that she is not a medical or scientific expert. She understands the objections that have been made against the vaccine's accelerated testing and deployment, but she also has every reason to believe that the public health authorities who approved the vaccine are competent and sincere. To what degree should she weigh the advice of experts against her own uncertainty?

Should Marlene report Rebecca and her family for their violation of isolation laws? Suppose the authorities charge Rebecca with violating quarantine. What degree of punishment (if any) is appropriate? Is the violation of quarantine or physical distancing laws a relatively minor offense, comparable to a traffic violation? Is it a more serious criminal offense, comparable to manslaughter? Explain.

QUESTIONS FOR REFLECTION

1. How should a state decide when to reopen during a pandemic? What prudential and moral values should guide this decision? What weight should be allotted to each value? Adjudicate between Friedersdorf and Caplan.

2. If we were to adopt Weinstock's suggestion to use more of the 24-hour day, would this cause inequities? For example, would all workers be asked to adopt this new schedule or would this fall disproportionately on low-wage "essential workers"? How would single parents meet their child-care needs on a 24-hour schedule?

3. Is it morally permissible for a state to mandate vaccinations? Does it matter whether the mandate is for children or adults? Would such a mandate need to allow for non-medical reasons to decline vaccination (e.g., religious objections or vaccine hesitancy)?

Permissions Acknowledgments

Caplan, Arthur. "The Price of Going Back to Work Too Soon." *The Hastings Centre Bioethics Forum*. 6 Apr 2020. Licensed under CC BY-ND 4.0. https://creativecommons.org/licenses/by-nd/4.0/.

Cegłowski, Maciej. "We Need a Massive Surveillance Program." *Idle Words Blog*. 23 Mar 2020. Copyright © 2020 Maciej Cegłowski. Reprinted with permission.

Douglas, Tom. "Flouting Quarantine." *Stockholm Centre Blog*. 24 Mar 2020. Reprinted with permission.

Emanuel, Ezekiel J., et al. "Fair Allocation of Scarce Medical Resources in the Time of Covid-19." *The New England Journal of Medicine* 382 (2020): 2049–55. Copyright © 2020 Massachusetts Medical Society. Reprinted with permission from Massachusetts Medical Society.

Eyal, Nir, Marc Lipsitch, and Peter Smith. "Human Challenge Studies to Accelerate Coronavirus Vaccine Licensure." *The Journal of Infectious Diseases* 221.11 (1 June 2020): 1752–56. Copyright © 2020 The Authors. Published by Oxford University Press for the Infectious Diseases Society of America. Reproduced with permission.

Fins, Joseph J. "Disabusing the Disability Critique of the New York State Task Force Report on Ventilator Allocation." *The Hastings Centre Bioethics Forum*. 1 Apr 2020. Licensed under CC BY-ND 4.0. https://creativecommons.org/licenses/by-nd/4.0/.

Folkers, Kelly McBride and Arthur Caplan. "False Hope about Coronavirus Treatments." *The Hastings Centre Bioethics Forum*. 20 Mar 2020. Licensed under CC BY-ND 4.0. https://creativecommons.org/licenses/by-nd/4.0/.

Friedersdorf, Conor. "Take the Shutdown Skeptics Seriously." *The Atlantic.com*. 7 Apr 2020. Copyright © 2020 The Atlantic. All rights reserved. Used under license.

Held, Shai. "The Staggering, Heartless Cruelty toward the Elderly." *The Atlantic.com*. 12 Mar 2020. Copyright © 2020 The Atlantic. All rights reserved. Used under license.

Holmes, Seth and Liza Buchbinder. "In a Defunded Health System, Doctors and Nurses Suffer Near-Impossible Conditions." *Salon.com*. 29 Mar 2020.

Kenny, Nuala P., Susan Sherwin, and Francoise E. Baylis. "Re-visioning Public Health Ethics: A Relational Perspective." *Canadian Journal of Public Health* 101.1 (Jan 2010): 9–11. Copyright © 2010. Reprinted by permission from Springer Nature via Copyright Clearance Center.

Lowe, Abbey, Angela Hewlett, and Toby Schonfeld. "How Should Clinicians Respond to International Public Health Emergencies?" *AMA Journal of Ethics* 22.1 (2020): 6–21. Used under the open access terms of AMA Journal of Ethics.

McDonald, Sean. "Coronavirus: A Digital Governance Emergency of International Concern." Opinion. *Cigionline.org.* 2 Mar 2020. Copyright © 2020 The Centre for International Governance Innovation. Reprinted with permission.

Miller, Franklin G. "Why I Support Age-Related Rationing of Ventilators for Covid-19 Patients." *The Hastings Centre Bioethics Forum.* 9 Apr 2020. Licensed under CC BY-ND 4.0. https://creativecommons.org/licenses/by-nd/4.0/.

Ossei-Owusu, Shaun. "Coronavirus and the Politics of Disposability." *Boston Review.net.* 8 Apr 2020. Reprinted with author's permission.

Savulescu, Julian. "Is It Right to Cut Corners in the Search for a Coronavirus Cure?" Opinion section. *The Guardian.com.* 25 Mar 2020. Copyright © 2020 Guardian News & Media Ltd.

Schuklenk, Udo. "Health Care Professionals Are under No Ethical Obligation to Treat COVID-19 Patients." *Journal of Medical Ethics Blog.* Ed. Hazem Zohny and Mike King. 1 Apr 2020. Copyright © 2020 BMJ. Used with permission of BMJ. All rights reserved.

Scully, Jackie Leach. "Disablism in a Time of Pandemic." *IJFAB Blog.* 1 Apr 2020. First published on the official IJFAB Blog. Reprinted with author's permission.

Skelton, Anthony and Lisa Forsberg. "Mandating Vaccination." Copyright © 2020 Anthony Skelton and Lisa Forsberg. Used with authors' permission.

Thompson, Derek. "The Technology that Could Free America from Quarantine." *The Atlantic.com.* 7 Apr 2020. Copyright © 2020 The Atlantic. All rights reserved. Used under license.

Weinstock, Daniel. "A Harm Reduction Approach to Physical Distancing." *Policy for Pandemics.* Newsletter. Issue 21 (21 Apr 2020). Reprinted with author's permission.

The publisher has made every attempt to locate all copyright holders of the material published in this book, and would be grateful for information that would allow correction of any errors or omissions in subsequent editions of the book.

Index

*Numbers in **bold** indicate where the term is defined.*

From the Publisher

A name never says it all, but the word "Broadview" expresses a good deal of the philosophy behind our company. We are open to a broad range of academic approaches and political viewpoints. We pay attention to the broad impact book publishing and book printing has in the wider world; for some years now we have used 100% recycled paper for most titles. Our publishing program is internationally oriented and broad-ranging. Our individual titles often appeal to a broad readership too; many are of interest as much to general readers as to academics and students.

Founded in 1985, Broadview remains a fully independent company owned by its shareholders—not an imprint or subsidiary of a larger multinational.

For the most accurate information on our books (including information on pricing, editions, and formats) please visit our website at www.broadviewpress.com. Our print books and ebooks are also available for sale on our site.

broadview press
www.broadviewpress.com

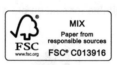